101 Tips on Getting into Medical School

Second Edition: Updated, Revised, Enlarged

This guide is a must-have for all medical school applicants! With her insider's view, Jennifer Welch offers realistic advice that makes the dreaded application process more clear, and honest tips to helping candidates avoid often fatal flaws. I wish I had had this when I applied to medical school!

Jason L. Freedman, M.D.
Hematology-Oncology
Children's Hospital of Philadelphia
Pediatrics
Columbia University Medical Center

This book provides a comprehensive and practical guide on how to navigate successfully the medical school application process. In addition to clarifying the many tangible requirements that are necessary to be competitive, Jennifer Welch gives the reader a window into the intangibles that significantly impact an admissions decision. An excellent read for both the savvy and the "clueless" medical school applicant.

Paula Jacobs
Senior Associate Director
Student and Career Development
College of Human Ecology
Cornell University

How will YOU stand out among the tens of thousands of students who apply to medical school each year? This guide takes you through the often overwhelming process of applying to medical school and shows you what schools and admissions committees are *really* looking for.

Using real-life scenarios from thousands of medical school applications and interviews, this second, updated, revised, and enlarged edition of *101 Tips* will teach you what works — and what does not! — from *inside* the admissions process.

Great advice — from choosing pre-med courses to wowing the interview committee — has been selected by those who have seen the process first-hand. This guide provides the best tips drawn from thousands of winning applicants, all from the perspective of a unique insider, a medical school admissions director.

The author, Jennifer C. Welch, M.S., is the Director of Admissions at the fifteenth oldest medical school in the United States.

101 TIPS

— on getting into —

MEDICAL SCHOOL

Jennifer C. Welch

Second Edition
Updated, Revised, Enlarged

≫ North Syracuse, New York ≪
≪ Gegensatz Press ≫
≫ 2009 ≪

Cataloging-in-Publication:

Welch, Jennifer C. (Jennifer Cox), 1971-
    101 tips on getting into medical school / Jennifer C. Welch.
        128 p. ; 23 cm.
        2nd ed., updated, revised, enlarged.
    "Jennifer C. Welch, M.S., is the Director of Admissions at the fifteenth
oldest medical school in the United States."
    ISBN 978-1-933237-28-2 (softcover)
    ISBN 978-1-933237-27-5 (e-book)
1. Medical colleges—United States—Admissions. 2. Medical colleges—United
States—Entrance requirements. 3. Premedical education—United States.
[DNLM: 1. Schools, Medical. 2. School Admission Criteria. 3. United States.
W 19 W439o 2009]
I. Title. II Title: One hundred and one tips on getting into medical school.
    R838.4 W44o 2009   610.71/173—dc22   AACR2
Library of Congress Control Number (1st ed.) 2006936128

Second edition, updated, revised, enlarged. Printed in the U.S.A.

The guillemets, or two pairs of opposing chevrons, dark on the lower cusps and
light on the upper, are a trademark of Gegensatz Press.

Distributed to the trade worldwide by:
Gegensatz Press
108 Deborah Lane
North Syracuse, NY 13212-1931
<www.gegensatzpress.com>

Cover by Sabra Snyder.
Photographs by Deborah Rexine.
Design by Eric v.d. Luft.

101 Tips on Getting into Medical School

Second Edition: Updated, Revised, Enlarged

Contents

About the Author

Jennifer Welch has worked in college admissions since 1993 and has advised thousands of students in preparing their applications to college. As a school counselor and a college admissions professional, she has been a successful liaison between prospective students and various academic institutions on both the secondary and collegiate levels.

Since 2001 she has served as Director of Admissions at the State University of New York (SUNY) Upstate Medical University, one of North America's oldest medical schools. In this capacity, she has guided thousands of prospective students through the entire application process, evaluated thousands of student applications, participated as a voting member on several admissions committees, visited hundreds of colleges and universities, and has developed successful recruitment strategies.

She received a bachelor of arts degree in economics from the SUNY College at Potsdam and a master of science degree in school counseling from Syracuse University. She lives in Marcellus, New York, with her husband, Dennis, and their three children.

Preface

This book is a basic "do's and don'ts" designed to provide applicants with an "inside" perspective on the medical school application and admission process. Too often applicants hurry or delay their applications or hurt their chances of admission by heeding the wrong advice, or making assumptions about what is or is not required or acceptable in the application process.

Prospective students should use this as a guide in preparing for the often overwhelming process of applying to medical school. It is not intended to be a comprehensive document; rather it provides a basic overview of the medical school admissions process. The book attempts to clarify that process and help students avoid some common mistakes that the author has seen time and time again. It is intended to provide real-world practical advice about how to navigate the complex medical college admissions process. While there are Web sites, books, and physicians that may be able to provide applicants with information and advice regarding the admissions process, few of these sources are actually able to speak from the inside point of view of an admissions director. These tips are based on years of first-hand experience from someone who has actively helped to set the standards for, and played an integral role in, selecting the incoming classes for a medical school.

The information provided here is by no means a guarantee of acceptance. For concrete information about a particular medical school, applicants should check directly with the admissions office at that school. Contact information for each medical school is listed in the back of this book.

Acknowledgments

This book would not have been possible without the knowledge, encouragement, mentoring, friendship, and vision of Dr. E. Gregory Keating, Dean of Student Affairs and Associate Dean of Admissions at SUNY Upstate Medical University, 2001-2006. We were looking forward to writing this book together until Greg's very untimely and tragic death in August 2006. No one was more dedicated to students and their success than Greg. Not a day goes by that I do not think about him and miss his humor, support, drive, positive attitude, his passion for life, and his work.

I am so thankful to my family for all their love and support while putting this book together. To my husband, thank you for listening to me and for your support. To my children, I love you to the moon and back — you are my inspiration and my life. To my parents, sisters, and sister-in-law, whose love, support, and encouragement got me here, thank you for all you do.

A very special thank you to Isabelle Rhoades, my close friend and colleague, for keeping me focused while writing this book. I am so appreciative for your feedback, ideas, editing assistance, comic relief, and most of all, your friendship. I could not have done this without you!

Thank you to Debbie Rexine for a great photo and Sabra Snyder for a fabulous cover design. You are both truly talented women.

Thank you to Candace Rhea and Julie Antoniou for all your editing assistance and help in making this book flow. I really appreciate all your efforts.

To Eric Luft, Ph.D., thank you for making this book come to life! I am not sure I would have gotten this far without you! Greg would have been proud that we were able to do this together.

To Carolyn Couch and Carol Morath, thank you both so much for taking such good care of me all these years. You make my job and life so much easier. Thank you to Donna Vavonese, Joni Hinds, Leah Caldwell, and Susan Stearns, Ph.D., for all your ideas, encouragement, honesty, and assistance!

To Lynn Cleary, M.D., Vice President for Academic Affairs, thank you for giving me the opportunity to put this book together and for the encouragement and feedback you have provided along the way.

To Julie R. White, Ph.D., Dean of Student Affairs, thank you for the encouragement and friendship you give me each and every day. You are an amazing mentor and friend.

Thank you to Joni Huff, Director of Admissions, Pritzker School of Medicine at the University of Chicago and previous pre-health advisor at Yale University, and Paula Jacobs, pre-health advisor at Cornell University, for taking the time to read the manuscript and provide me with such valuable feedback. It is great to have such wonderful colleagues who are as dedicated to students and as passionate as you are about seeing students succeed in the health professions.

To Scott Cameron, M.D., Ph.D.; Nikki Gero, M.D., M.B.A.; Cameron Hall, M.D.; Joshua Nelson, MSIII; TeSha English, MSIII; and Jason Freedman, M.D. — thank you so much for taking the time out of your incredibly busy schedules to help me with this book.

Two authoritative Web sites furnished me with extensive and substantial data: the AAMC page on "Facts — Applicants, Matriculants, and Graduates: MCAT Scores and GPAs for Applicants and Matriculants to U.S. Medical Schools, 1997-2008" <www.aamc.org/data/facts/2008/ 2008mcatgpa.htm>, used for Tip 20; and the E-Zine at CollegeGrad.com. "The Most Important Interview Non-Verbals." <www.collegegrad.com/ezine/ 21nonver.shtml>, quoted in Tip 92.

This book is dedicated to the memory of E. Gregory Keating, Ph.D. I could not have asked for a better mentor, supervisor, or friend.

Getting Ready

The following information is for prospective medical students to use as a general guideline in the application and admissions process for medical school. Each undergraduate college may do things a little differently, so it is important for you to seek out the resources that are available to you on your campus. Your pre-health advisor will play a key role in helping you prepare for this huge undertaking. Make sure you work closely with him or her. It is best to meet with your advisor early and regularly and to take advantage of all that he or she has to offer.

1. Be aware of all the reasons why you are interested in a medical career.

You must be confident that a medical career is something you are deeply committed to, and you must be able to convey that commitment both verbally and in writing. Simply saying that you have always wanted to be a physician because you want to "help people" or that you enjoy watching *House* or *Grey's Anatomy* will not be enough. Spend some time really thinking about all the reasons why you are doing this, and be sure that your reasons are thoughtful, clear, and true to the person you are.

If you are convinced that medical school is the right career path for you, be sure that you are doing it for all the "right" reasons. You need to know exactly what you are getting yourself into. You will eventually need to convince medical school admissions committees that you are genuinely motivated to pursue a career in medicine.

Be sure that you can answer the "Why medicine?" question. Again, simply answering, "Because I want to help people," will not be enough. There are many careers that help people. You need to be able to articulate the reasons you are choosing medicine instead of deciding to be a physician assistant, nurse, physical therapist, medical radiographer, social worker, or biology teacher.

Actions speak louder than words. In addition to being able to articulate clearly your decision and aptitude for a career in medicine, keep in mind this old adage and take the time to gain exposure to and learn about the field to which you hope someday to contribute and in which you hope to be a part. The importance of getting relevant clinical experience will be emphasized throughout both this book and the application process. More than anything, clinical experience will benefit you as you try to answer and convey "Why medicine?" first to yourself and then to others. Apart from having all the right words and good intentions, it is impossible to know truly that medicine is the right path for you, or to convince an interviewer or committee of this, until you have taken the time to experience it and see the good, the bad, and the ugly that comes along with being a physician. If medicine is indeed the right career choice for you, clinical experience should give you more specific reasons for wanting to become a doctor. It will also enable you to share with your interviewers particular instances and experiences of observing doctors and interacting with patients. This will carry more weight than merely having good intentions.

Getting into medical school is not easy. Less than half the students who apply to medical school each year are accepted. Medical schools are looking for the most intelligent and motivated students they can find. Successful applicants will need to demonstrate a clear desire to work with and help people, will need to work hard, and will need to be committed to the field of medicine.

2. Be realistic about your chances for admission.

A 2.0 cumulative grade point average (GPA) and a single-digit combined Medical College Admissions Test (MCAT) score will not get you into medical school. Take the time to research thoroughly the schools to which you plan to apply and be realistic about your chances of gaining admission to them, or to any medical school. Research your target medical schools' average MCAT test scores and GPAs. Many schools have this information available on their Web sites. Contact information for each medical school is listed at the end of this book.

Medical College Admission Test (MCAT)
www.aamc.org/mcat

The MCAT Care Team
Association of American Medical Colleges
Section for Applicant Assessment Services
2450 N Street, NW
Washington, DC 20037
Phone: (202) 828-0690

Most U.S. medical schools require applicants to submit MCAT scores. The MCAT is broken down into four different categories: Verbal Reasoning, Physical Sciences, Writing Sample, and Biological Sciences. The highest score that you can obtain in each of the Verbal Reasoning, Physical Science, and Biological Science areas is 15. The Writing Sample is scored using an alpha system, with the lowest score of "J" and the highest of "T."

Purchase the current edition of the *Medical School Admissions Requirements (MSAR)* book that is put together each year by the Association of American Medical Colleges (AAMC), because GPA and MCAT averages may change from year to year. Your pre-health advisor may also have a copy of this book for you to use as a reference.

> **Association of American Medical Colleges (AAMC)**
> *www.aamc.org/students*
>
> *The AAMC has very useful reference tools as you begin the medical school application process. The Web site contains information on each medical school, contact information, various publications, student responsibility information, medical school responsibility information, tips on applying to medical school, financial planning information, information for minority students, and health professions advisor information.*

3. Visit with your pre-med advisor often and early.

If you are currently in college, it is very important to maintain close contact with your pre-health or pre-med advisor. A mistake that many students make in this process is either not meeting with him or her at all, or meeting with him or her too late. Your pre-health advisor is an invaluable resource and should be sought out early in your college career. He or she will be very helpful in assisting you through this rather daunting experience. Be sure that you have a good working relationship with your advisor, and be sure to take his or her advice seriously. In many cases, your advisor will be the person responsible for providing your letter(s) of recommendation to medical schools. If you have a solid relationship with your advisor, he or she can provide a letter from someone who knows you well and can comment on your character, ambition, and suitability for a career in medicine. This more personal letter will be more effective than one simply stating that the writer has had one appointment with you, that you arrived on time, and that you were pleasant and attentive during the meeting.

Keep in mind that most schools have a process for requesting a pre-health committee letter. Depending on the school, the process can be quite lengthy and may involve scheduling an appointment several months in advance, a subsequent interview, soliciting letters from various professors on your behalf, a composite write-up of your interview, a summary of the letters submitted on your behalf by professors, and the committee's overall recommendation. All this takes time. Medical schools are aware of which colleges and universities have pre-health advisors or committees available. If you do not submit a pre-health letter because you waited until the last minute to request one, or did not ask for one, this could be viewed as a "red flag." The committee will most likely question why you did not submit a letter from your pre-health advisor or committee and may make the assumption that you procrastinated or failed to do so to avoid receiving an unfavorable recommendation.

If there is no pre-health advisor on your campus or if you are a non-traditional student, the National Association of Advisors for the Health Professionals (NAAHP) advisor-at-large service may be able to provide you with some advice on applying to medical school. Its Web site <www.naahp.org> provides a list of members willing to volunteer their time to help applicants who do not have access to an advisor. There is also a list of colleges and universities that do have health professions advisors available on their campus.

4. Applying to medical school is a very long process.

Be prepared! You must begin the application process more than a year in advance of the year in which you hope to matriculate. A general timeline for traditional applicants might look something like this:

Freshman Year

Meet your pre-health advisor.
Get involved in student run pre-health (or pre-med) clubs or groups.
Get off to a good start academically.
Begin extracurricular activities.
Look into opportunities for a medically related summer job or
        volunteer experience.

Summer Courses

It is best for students to complete medical school prerequisites during the academic year at the undergraduate college or university where they are enrolled. If you must take summer courses to complete your degree or complete another major, be sure you do so at a similar type of college as the one where you are matriculated. Completing science courses during the summer is generally not recommended.

Sophomore Year

Maintain contact with your pre-health advisor.
Attend any medically related pre-health events or activities on your
        campus.
Maintain a solid academic record, by doing well and taking
        academically challenging courses each semester.
Continue your extracurricular involvement.
Get involved in research opportunities, if they interest you.
Look into opportunities for a medically related summer job or
        volunteer experience.
Look into participating in a summer medical careers program.
Begin looking into the different medical schools. This is a good
        time to purchase a copy of the *MSAR*.

Medical School Admissions Requirements (MSAR) Book

This is a "must-have" book. It has invaluable information on each participating medical school, including:

> *Deadlines and requirements.*
> *The average GPAs and MCAT scores of matriculated students.*
> *Contact information for each medical school.*
> *Financial aid information, including tuition costs and special program information.*

Purchase a copy of the MSAR at <www.aamc.org/publications>, or ask your pre-health advisor if you can borrow a copy.

Junior Year

Continue to maintain a strong academic record.
Complete all medical school prerequisite requirements.
Continue your extracurricular involvement.
Meet with your pre-health advisor regularly.
Select your letter of recommendation writers.
Interview with the pre-health committee.
Prepare for the MCATs.
Take the MCAT exam in the spring or early summer.
Familiarize yourself with the different application services:
- American Medical College Application Service (AMCAS)
- Texas Medical and Dental Schools Application Service (TMDSAS)
- American Association of Colleges of Osteopathic Medicine Application Service (AACOMAS).

American Medical College
Application Service (AMCAS)
www.aamc.org/amcas

2450 N Street, NW
Washington, DC 20037-1126
Phone: (202) 828-0600
E-mail: amcas@aamc.org

AMCAS is a centralized processing center for first-year
applicants at participating allopathic (regular) medical
schools in the United States. Please see the end of this book
for those schools currently participating in AMCAS.

Summer Between
Junior and Senior Year

Complete a medically related summer job or volunteer
        experience.
Participate in a summer medical careers program.
Narrow down the list of medical schools that you will be
        applying to.
Submit your application and all your college transcripts to
        AMCAS.
Request that your letters of recommendation be sent to your pre-
        health office.
Let your pre-health office know which schools you are applying
        to and where your letters of recommendation should be
        sent.
Take the MCATs, if you have not already.
Complete any secondary applications you receive.

Texas Medical and Dental Schools
Application Service (TMDSAS)
www.utsystem.edu/tmdsas

702 Colorado, Suite 6.400
Austin, TX 78701
Phone: (512) 499-4785

TMDSAS is a centralized processing center for students applying to the seven allopathic medical schools in Texas. Please see the end of this book for the schools currently participating in TMDSAS.

American Association of Colleges of Osteopathic
Medicine Application Service (AACOMAS)
aacomas.aacom.org

5550 Friendship Boulevard
Suite 310
Chevy Chase, MD 20815-7231
Phone: (301) 968-4190
E-mail: aacomas@aacom.org

AACOMAS is the centralized processing center for students applying to twenty-seven of the twenty-eight osteopathic (D.O.) medical schools in the United States. There are twenty-five colleges of osteopathic medicine and three branch campuses.

Fall of Senior Year

Finish any outstanding secondary applications.
Make sure that your applications are complete at each of the
        medical schools.
Interview at medical schools.
Continue to maintain a strong academic record.
Continue your extracurricular involvement.

Spring of Senior Year

Continue to maintain a strong academic record.
Begin looking into financial resources.
Submit the Free Application for Federal Student Aid form (FAFSA)
        <www.fafsa.ed.gov>.
Attend Second Visit Days to help narrow down your choices.
Finish the degree program you are enrolled in.
Make your final decision on which medical school you will attend,
        and withdraw from the others no later than May 15.

Multiple Acceptance Day
May 15

*If you are fortunate enough to be accepted at multiple
schools, it is important to release other acceptances as
soon as you know where you will be attending medical
school. In fairness to the many other qualified applicants
waiting for openings at the various medical schools, there
is no reason for students to be holding on to seven or eight
acceptances at any given time. After May 15, medical
schools may rescind an acceptance to applicants who are
holding more than one medical school acceptance.*

> ### *Criminal Background Check Information*
> *www.aamc.org/students/amcas/faq/background.htm*
>
> *The AAMC has started a national background check service for applicants once they are accepted. This service has been initiated so that medical schools can receive appropriate national criminal histories, and to avoid applicants having to pay additional fees at each medical school to which they are accepted.*

Summer after Senior Year

Send final transcripts to the medical school you will be attending.
Attend orientation program.
Begin medical school!

5. Applying to medical school can be a very expensive process.

During a one-year application cycle, you could spend between $3,500 and $5,000 just to apply to medical school:

> AMCAS application fees. AMCAS processing fess are $160 for the first medical school application and $31 for each medical school thereafter.
> Secondary application fees ($45-$100 each).
> Travel expenses (airfare, bus or train, taxis, parking).
> Hotel costs (one or two nights depending on distance and length of interview day).

Interview clothes.
Food.
Other incidentals.

The Number of Applications for Medical School

The number of medical schools that a student applies to will vary, but many applicants each apply to fifteen or twenty different medical schools. The AAMC data reports that the average number of applications per applicant for the last few years was twelve to thirteen. Keep in mind that there are a number of students who apply Early Decision (ED) or to other special programs where they will only apply to one medical school.

---

6. Dare to be different. Stand out in the application process!

There are far too many "cookie cutter" applicants who all look the same on paper and in black interview suits. You need to set yourself apart from all the other applicants.

Figure out what is special about you and what you have to offer the field of medicine that sets you apart from all the other applicants. Get involved in a variety of quality activities and when you find something that you love, stick with it. Participate in activities because you really want to and because you enjoy them, not because they will look good on your resumé. You will easily be able to convey your enthusiasm for activities and experiences about which you are passionate, but not for activities that you took part in because you thought you had to do them in order to get into medical school.

7. Major in whatever you want.

While it is true that the majority of applicants to medical school are or were science majors, you do not **have** to major in biology or chemistry. There are many other fascinating fields of study available: psychology, theatre arts, history, computer science, English, etc. If you are interested in a particular program of study, pursue it!

Other majors will provide you with a different perspective on the field of medicine and could be looked upon very favorably by an admissions committee. Be careful about trying to impress medical schools by choosing programs of study that are viewed as more difficult, such as neuroscience or biophysics. If the result is a much lower GPA, the admissions committee may doubt your ability to be successful in the basic science years of your medical school education.

It is much easier to do well in a subject or major that you enjoy versus one that you chose because of its rigorous reputation. Challenge yourself, but make sure you major in something that interests you and that you enjoy studying. Medical schools are also striving for diversity in their classes and students with backgrounds other than biology or chemistry can often contribute interesting perspectives to class discussions, ethics issues, etc.

8. Find a balance in your life.

You will need to juggle your academics, personal life, extracurricular activities, family, and personal time while in medical school. Study hard, get involved, investigate the field of medicine, and love what you do.

Many people entering a health profession are combining their vocation and their avocation; they make their work their play. You will truly need to love this job. There will be many long and difficult days, and you must be passionate about what you are getting into. Having a good balance of work and play will help you to find release from the stress that you may end up facing on a daily basis.

It is very important for you to find this balance. It will help you to be successful, not only in medical school, but also in your career.

9. Let the admissions office know if you are applying during the same application year as your husband, wife, or significant other.

Be sure to let the medical schools to which you are applying know this early in the application cycle. Most medical schools are willing to cluster your interview schedules, making it easier for both you and the school. This will allow you the opportunity possibly to save money and time, and ultimately may help in making your decision on where to attend medical school.

10. Consider taking some time off between college and medical school.

Taking time off from academics before entering medical school is becoming more common, and it occurs for a variety of reasons: research opportunities, clinical experiences, traveling abroad, and family or financial reasons, such as working to pay off undergraduate student loans. It also may be a good time for you to decide if the medical profession is the right career for you. Medical schools are seeing more and more non-traditional applicants, including students who have been out of school for a while or who may be changing careers. Many of these applicants wanted to be physicians earlier in their lives, but felt it was unattainable. Only now are they realizing that they should have followed their hearts from the beginning.

It is very important to not rush this process. Too often, applicants are in a hurry to apply, because of the long application cycle, and do so without taking the time necessary to submit the best application possible. These applicants often end up being denied and ultimately have to start the process over again.

Medical schools want you to apply when you are ready. For some applicants that is right out of college, but for others it is after years of pursuing another career, taking time to reflect, or starting a family. Be prepared to articulate clearly why you took time off or why you decided to change careers.

Applying to
Medical School

The application that you submit to medical schools must be perfect! Spend a great deal of time putting it together. Everything that you submit in the application will be looked at and evaluated. Spell words correctly, use proper grammar, and punctuate appropriately.

Keep in mind that there will be many people reviewing your application. Members of the admissions committee may have very different backgrounds or perspectives about potential medical school students, and they may not all be looking for the same things in your application. Some may value your clinical experiences more highly and others may be more interested in the courses that you took and the grades that you received.

It is also important not to think of applying to medical school as simply a checklist. ("If I do this, this, and this, then I will be accepted into medical school.") Every applicant is looked at as an individual. The admissions committee is hoping to find something different in each and every applicant. They often ask, "What can this student contribute to the field of medicine that is different from everyone else?"

With extracurricular activities, quality matters more than quantity. Choose activities that are meaningful to you. Your activities should reflect your personal and academic interests, and allow you to demonstrate qualities such as initiative, ability to handle responsibility, leadership skills, critical thinking skills, and a commitment to service work in your community. Meaningful experiences are a must.

A medical school education is among the most standardized types of education offered. All students need to learn the same material and pass the board and licensing exams in order to practice medicine. Apply to and attend a medical school that will offer you what you are looking for in a medical education, one where you think you will be happy and fit in, and that will provide the best experience possible for you. You are more likely to do well and thrive in an environment that meets both your academic and your social needs.

> ### *What Medical Schools Look For In an Applicant*
>
> *Academic achievement.*
> *Meaningful experiences dealing with and relating to people.*
> > *Extracurricular activities.*
> > *Service volunteer work.*
> > *Clinical experience.*
> *Character.*
> *Drive and motivation for a career in medicine.*
> > *Personal statement.*
> > *Interview — communication skills.*

11. Apply early!

Medical school admission is very competitive, so you must get your applications in **early**. Schools with rolling admissions review their applications as they come in. As students are accepted, there will be more and more competition for the smaller number of remaining spots available. Admissions committees will then have a greater number of other applicants to compare with you for those few remaining seats. You are, in a sense, stacking the odds against yourself by procrastinating.

The AMCAS application process begins every year on or around May 1, and applicants may begin filling out their applications at that time. Approximately June 1 of each year is the first day that applicants may submit their applications to AMCAS.

It is not in your best interest to wait until right before a medical school's deadline to apply. Here's why: If you apply to a medical school on November 1 (the AMCAS deadline for the medical school that you are applying to), you will meet that deadline, but if the medical school has a final deadline for a completed application of December 1, you may not make the medical school's own deadline for having a completed application on file. AMCAS is very clear that it may take four to six weeks to verify an application — and that is if everything goes smoothly. It is not uncommon for additional information to be requested, delaying the verification of your initial AMCAS application and, in turn, delaying your application from being received or reviewed by the medical schools of your choice. Clearly, it is not in an applicant's best interest to wait until the very last day to apply to medical school. You will not be able to meet the medical school's final deadline.

This is also true of schools that do not have rolling admission, such as Harvard, Yale, or Johns Hopkins. It is always in your best interest to apply early, when more interview positions are available.

While application deadline extensions can be requested, they are rarely granted and are usually requested as a result of procrastination on the applicant's part. To avoid the complication of requesting an extension, start the application process early and be proactive. Keep in mind the kind of impression you are making on the admissions committee when you have to request additional time in order to complete your application. Enrolling in medical school and later becoming a physician requires a great deal of responsibility, organization, and time management. Your inability to meet a deadline for which you have been allotted ample time might speak volumes about how you will perform in the future, as a student, and eventually as a physician.

12. If you call the admissions office, always ask with whom you are speaking, write down his or her name, the date of your call, and the reason for your call.

If you need permission to deviate from the stated policies, be sure you know to whom you are speaking and mark the date and time. It is important to follow-up with an e-mail confirming what you were told. If, for example, your application was late and you called to get an extension, you must be able to verify that a deadline extension was granted by someone in the admissions office. Another example might be that students will sometimes contact an admissions office to have a course evaluated or to determine whether or not they have successfully met one of the required prerequisite courses for admission. While most admissions offices keep a record of such requests and decisions, considering the amount of e-mails and the volume of mail received each day, things do get lost or misplaced, despite best efforts. It is important to keep a record of such exceptions and decisions, to keep track of which schools granted their approval and which did not. In case the issue should come up again, you will have documentation of the decision.

13. Include everything in your application that you really want the admissions committee to know about you.

It is important for the admissions committee to know if you have experience working with the elderly, volunteering at a boys' and girls' club, or shadowing a doctor while you were in high school. These experiences tell the committee that your interest in serving others has been ongoing. As a physician, you will be dedicating your life to serving other people. It is important that you have evidence of this dedication in your application. Even an experience such as waiting on tables shows that you have had experience managing your time, dealing with difficult people, and multitasking. These demonstrated skills are important and all say something about you as an applicant.

Include all clinically related or volunteer experiences in the activities section of your application, even if you mention them in your personal statement. It is perfectly acceptable to describe an experience there and also to mention it later in your personal statement. If an admissions officer is scanning your application during an initial review, these relevant experiences may be very easily overlooked. List the experiences. Make them easily identifiable and very clear. Do not make an admissions person search for them. That could make a difference in the outcome of your application.

Elements of a Good Application

Imagine the reader.
Be perfect in grammar.
Have no typos.
Be succinct.
Be understated.
Be honest.

---

14. Do not leave it up to the admissions committee to decide why your grades were so poor during a particular semester.

If your grades were weak during a particular semester or year, it is important that you address this somewhere in your application or in a letter to the admissions committee.

Do not leave it to up to the admissions committee to determine what was going on in your life during that time. The committee will notice the inconsistency in your grades.
They will wonder whether you are trying to hide something, and may question your ability to perform consistently well academically. Do not make excuses about what was going on, just be honest and straightforward.

Admissions committees look for a progression of grades. They want to be sure that, as you take more challenging courses each year, your GPA continues to rise. When evaluating applications, in an effort to select students for their next incoming class, the admissions committee wants to be assured that if you are accepted, you will consistently work hard and be successful in medical school. If there was any extenuating circumstance that affected your academic performance, such as an illness or the loss of a close family member, share this information.

15. Make sure that you have a professional contact e-mail address.

E-mail addresses such as <drgoodluv@hotmail.com>, <imastud247@yahoo.com>, or <Qteepie@gmail.com> are inappropriate to use when applying to medical school. Addresses such as these can tell an admissions committee a lot about your character that you may not even realize. Always put forth your most professional side when communicating with an admissions office. You never know what they are looking at and how you are being evaluated.

16. If you have a page on Facebook, MySpace, or YouTube, make sure that it is professional.

Attending medical school is just the first professional step in the process of becoming a physician. You need to act in a professional way from the beginning of the application process. Sites like Facebook, MySpace, or YouTube can be a great way to stay in touch with friends, but as with all things, you **never** want to put anything on these sites that could reflect a less-than-professional aspect of your personality. It is a **very** small world. Be mindful of this, and of any images or information that you put out on these social networking sites. Admissions committees may not have time to look at these sites for every applicant, but more and more schools are researching prospective students online to see what other information is available, in addition to whatever you may have submitted to them in your formal application.

17. Do not inundate the admissions committee with supplemental materials.

Admissions committee members do not have the time to review supplemental materials, such as CDs, videos, DVDs, portfolios, or three-ring binders. In most cases, you are welcome to send a brief update indicating an abstract, information on a recent publication, new clinical experiences, or something special that you have accomplished, but do not send volumes of new information. Chances are that it will not be reviewed.

18. Be careful how you treat all members of the admissions office staff.

Be polite and pleasant to all your contacts in the admissions office. Do not argue with any of them under any circumstances. If you are rude or inconsiderate to the support or clerical staff, it may get back to the admissions director or the admissions committee, and could have damaging effects on your candidacy for admission. Remember, how you present yourself says something about how, as a physician, you will interact with your patients, colleagues, and office personnel.

19. Do not inundate the admissions office with repeated phone calls.

When you must call to ask a question, trust that the answer is correct. You are dealing with admissions professionals who each follow their own medical school's policy and answer many of the same questions every day. If you have a concrete reason to be skeptical of the response that you are getting from the staff, ask to speak to the director.

     Use common sense. Calling the admissions office every day will probably work against you.

20. Be realistic about the number of schools that you apply to.

It is appropriate to apply to fifteen to twenty medical schools, but select them carefully. Talk to your pre-health advisor or use the *MSAR* to see which schools are the best for you to apply to, based on location, grades, test scores, type of teaching, tuition, and any other factors that are important to you.

It is also important to consider applying to a wide range of schools. You might be surprised to be rejected from a school where your GPA and MCAT scores are higher than its average. On the other hand, one of your "reach" schools might see something unique about you or your application and accept you. A good mix might be to apply to both state schools and private schools where your statistics are competitive, and also to one or two "reach" schools. Stay away from applying to schools outside your home state if they only accept two or three out-of-state applicants per year.

According to the AAMC, 42,231 people applied to medical school for the 2008 entering class. 18,036 accepted students (42.7% of applicants) ended up enrolling at one of the 129 U.S. allopathic medical schools that then existed.

Applicants and Matriculants to
U.S. Allopathic Medical Schools
AAMC Statistics on the 2008 Entering Class

Average overall GPA of applicants: 3.50
Average science GPA of applicants: 3.40
Average MCAT of applicants: 28.1 (P)

Average overall GPA of matriculants: 3.66
Average science GPA of matriculants: 3.60
Average MCAT of matriculants: 30.9 (P)

21. Take challenging courses.

Challenge yourself! Admissions committees take into consideration which courses you take and how you position them. Be sure to discuss course selections with your pre-health advisor. You want to take challenging courses each semester, preferably two science courses, each with a lab, and other challenging coursework. Be sure to take full course loads each semester and be careful not to add a lot of "fluff" courses. Earning a 3.7 for a semester in which you carried a full course load including several upper-level science courses will almost always carry more weight than a 3.9 earned for a semester when you took one rigorous science course surrounded by "fluff" courses like jazzercise or introduction to origami. It is really important to challenge yourself and to prove to the admissions committee that you can handle a rigorous academic course load.

22. Do not blame your professors for your poor grades.

Do not try to make excuses for your poor grades or try to defend them. If you are invited for an interview, be prepared to discuss those grades, but instead of placing the blame on someone else, focus on the positive and perhaps highlight your academic performance since then. Emphasize what you learned from the experience, such as adjusting your study habits, taking advantage of office hours, curtailing your extracurricular activities, or learning to manage your time better.

Even in medical school, you may have an instructor whose teaching style does not match your learning style, and you may need to learn the material on your own in order to succeed. Berating a professor or maligning his or her character or English speaking ability will not win you any points with your admissions interviewer. Not all professors are equally effective in the classroom and not all material is equally interesting to students. This is a reality in every academic setting.

You should present yourself as a person who is committed to achieving goals without blaming others when you encounter difficulties. This also speaks to how you will approach the heavy course load and different teaching styles within a medical institution.

23. Do not make excuses for poor MCAT scores.

Right after the MCAT scores are released, phones go wild in medical school admissions offices. It will not help to panic over disappointing scores, or to call or e-mail blaming your scores on "bad sushi" the day of the exam. Take responsibility for your disappointing scores, and be honest with yourself and the medical schools you are applying to.

If your scores are considerably lower than average, it may be necessary to retake the exam. However, applicants need to be aware that taking the MCAT multiple times could have a negative impact on their applications, unless there is a dramatic change in the scores. Though there is no longer a rule against repeating the MCATs more than three times, doing so will probably work against you.

It is also important to know how medical schools are looking at your MCAT scores. Though some medical schools may average your test scores or take the highest score in each subtest, most consider your most recent test scores the most important in the application process.

Keep in mind that most schools will only accept MCAT scores that are less than three years old, and there are some medical schools that will only accept them if they are less than two years old. Do your homework!

24. Know how to overcome a low GPA or MCAT score.

GPA and MCAT scores are usually the first items that an admissions committee looks at when evaluating a student's application. Grades and MCATs combined may carry 65% to 70% of the weight in the admissions decision. Admissions committees want to be sure that, if you are accepted, you will be successful academically in medical school and ultimately on your National Boards. The National Board exams are taken at the conclusion of the second and during the fourth year of medical school. MCATs play a bigger role in the admissions decision now that students are required to take shelf exams during their clerkship years. MCATs have proved to be a positive predictor of a student's ability to pass these exams.

Be sure that you have completed all the medical school prerequisites prior to sitting for the MCAT. The MCATs are offered many different times over the course of the year, so do not feel pressured to take them until you are ready. In April of the junior year, students are normally finishing either physics II or organic chemistry II, preparing for finals in all their other courses, getting ready to apply to medical school, and studying for the MCAT. Take your time and think about taking the May, June, or even the July exams. That will give you the opportunity to finish your course work, take your final exams, and then have adequate time to study for the MCATs without either feeling so much pressure to do it all at once or sacrificing your spring semester grades.

If you know that you have difficulty with standardized tests, or if you perform poorly the first time you take the MCATs, consider taking an MCAT prep course through Kaplan or the Princeton Review. Often, however, time and financial restraints prevent routine enrollment in MCAT prep courses.

If your MCAT scores are not what you had hoped, try to pinpoint your area of weak performance, but do not focus exclusively on that area as you prepare to take the exam again. You may need to bring your Verbal Reasoning scores up, but this should not be at the expense of Biological Science or Physical Science.

Try to stay balanced in preparing for the exam.

If your GPA, particularly your science GPA, is not as high as it should or could be to apply to medical school, or if your grades fluctuated greatly over the course of your college career, consider completing a master's degree in the hard sciences before applying to medical school. There are several one-year master's programs that you might want to consider. For instance, the programs at Boston University, Georgetown University, and the Johns Hopkins University all have a reputation for preparing students well for the medical school curriculum. These programs allow students to take medical school courses with current medical students and provide the pre-med students enrolled in these special master's programs with very good medical school advising.

Other strong "record enhancing" programs are at Drexel University and Duquesne University. Applicants looking to address a lower GPA are not limited to these programs. Any graduate program offering a master's degree in the sciences would be a possibility. Discuss your options with your pre-health advisor. There are also special programs designed for students underrepresented in medicine, such as Southern Illinois University's Medical/Dental Education Preparatory Program (MEDPREP).

If you came late to the decision to enter medical school or did not take the science prerequisites as an undergraduate, look for a postbaccalaureate program designed to give students interested in medicine the prerequisite courses they will need to apply to medical school. Check out the AAMC's postbaccalaureate premedical programs search engine at <www.services.aamc.org/postbac> for information on various programs. There are programs available that focus on applicants making a career change, applicants who need to enhance their academic records, minority applicants, and economically or educationally disadvantaged applicants.

25. Do not apply to medical school just because your parents want you to.

This may seem obvious, but medical school has to be **your** dream. Do not apply because of cultural pressure or because your mother or father wanted to become a doctor but could not.

Everyone understands familial pressure, but you have to really want this for yourself! If you are not completely open, honest, and passionate about pursuing a career in medicine, it is going to be a very long, hard road. If your disingenuous pursuit of medicine does not come through during your interview, it will come through within the first couple of years of medical school when your true interests will clash with the time and pressures of your courses. Medical school is a tremendous gift to those who attend and comes at great expense in time and money. Likewise, every person who serves at the medical school is dedicated to seeing students succeed in their pursuit. Medical school personnel invest in every way possible: with personal commitment, time, and money. Do not take this leap if you have any doubts. You need to do it only if **you** are passionate about it.

26. Be very careful when expressing any real or perceived personal connections during the admissions process.

Saying things like "Do you know who my father/mother is?" may not have the effect for which you had hoped. The process of applying, being accepted, and ultimately going to medical school is an independent process. You need to present yourself as an independent entity with the ability to obtain admission on your own, without acting as the child of Dr. ____. Your own ability to express yourself as an individual will make a more positive impression on those who are reviewing your record.

Eventually you will need to make quick decisions without relying on your friends or relations. Chances are, your father or mother is not going to be there when you have a life-or-death decision to make about one of your future patients.

27. Do not have your parents call to check on the status of your application.

By the time you apply to medical school, you really should be an independent student, doing things for yourself. Even if you think you do not have the time — make the time. It does not look good to an admissions committee when you cannot call on your own behalf to inquire about how your medical school application is progressing. For reasons of confidentiality, the admissions staff will not release information about your application or discuss the status of your application with your parents or spouse at any time anyway. Having them call on your behalf reflects badly on you and could ultimately have a negative impact on your candidacy.

28. Check with each medical school about its requirements, as each medical school may have different prerequisites.

Check with each medical school or take a look at the *MSAR* to see what courses each school requires for admission. Most require the basic pre-medical courses:

General biology I and II with lab
General chemistry I and II with lab
General physics I and II with lab (some may require
    calculus-based physics)
Organic chemistry I and II with lab
English courses

Other medical schools may require calculus, statistics, biochemistry, humanities, or social science courses.

Take some additional courses that may help you during your basic science years. These may include physiology, cell or molecular biology, histology, biochemistry, or genetics. They will be helpful in providing you with a solid foundation when completing your first two years of medical school.

Course work in the humanities, public health, the social sciences, expository writing, and ethics are also encouraged. Physicians must have strong interpersonal and communication skills and must be able to express their thoughts and ideas clearly. They also must have strong decision-making skills, be able to think independently, and be able to read and understand scientific articles.

Some medical schools do not have specific prerequisites, but recommend many of the above courses for students to be successful both in the first two years of medical school and on the MCATs.

Complete all your medical school prerequisites prior to submitting your application. Although this may not be required, preference may be given to those applicants who have completed all their prerequisites.

29. Do not assume that you can substitute AP or IB credits for your medical school prerequisites.

Check with each medical school regarding its Advanced Placement (AP) or International Baccalaureate (IB) policies. Some medical schools will not accept AP or IB credits to meet any of their medical school prerequisites. Other medical schools may accept the credits, but only if your primary undergraduate college has given you transfer credit and the courses are clearly indicated on your primary college transcript. Some medical schools may require that you take additional upper-level courses at your primary college in the subject area in which your AP or IB credit was earned in order to show that you can handle more rigorous college-level science courses.

     Also, if you want to substitute courses that you have taken for the medical school prerequisite courses (e.g., biochemistry in place of organic chemistry), you will need to check with each individual medical school to see which substitutions it will accept, if any. Medical school policies on course substitutions vary significantly.

30. Never assume that your application is complete.

Be proactive! It is your responsibility to be sure that all your application materials are received by the medical school's deadlines. Because of the volume of mail that admissions offices receive, it is best for you to follow up and confirm that each office has everything it needs and that items have arrived on time to complete your application.

     Do not assume anything or rely on the medical school

admissions office to notify you of an incomplete application or problems. By the time you learn what you are missing, it might be too late. Many schools have "applicant status" pages on their Web sites that provide an easy way for you to check to see if your application is complete and to track when materials arrive.

31. Keep your contact information current.

If any of your contact information changes over the course of the admissions process, be sure to update it with AMCAS and with each medical school.

If you are going to pay the money and go through the process of applying, you will want to make sure that you can be reached by the admissions staff if they try to contact you. Make sure that all schools have your correct phone number, current address, and correct e-mail address on file.

Be sure to let AMCAS know of your changes as well so that AMCAS and the schools you are applying to have consistent and correct contact information. Try not to invite confusion at any level of the application process.

32. Be a well-rounded applicant.

There are many different people on an admissions committee. It is important to keep in mind that each person is looking for something different in your application. That is the beauty of a committee. Some people are looking for students who have spent a great deal of time obtaining clinical experiences, others might be more interested in your research experiences, others in your grades and MCAT scores, and still others in your extracurricular activities during your undergraduate studies.

Your high school counselors probably told you that it was important to get involved and be a well-rounded applicant when applying to undergraduate colleges. Now you are hearing it again as you apply to medical school. Once you get to medical school your advisors are going to tell you the same thing in preparation for applying to residency programs. It is very important to get involved!

Admissions committees are eager to see applicants who have something more to offer the student body and the greater community than just good grades. They want to see significant contributions made both inside and outside the academic arena. They want to see that you will make a difference in the field of medicine.

Letters of Recommendation

Letters of recommendation can be one of the more stressful parts of completing an application, but they can also be one of the most important. Select your letter writers carefully and thoughtfully. Ask individuals who know you well and have insight into your intellectual capabilities and your interpersonal strengths. They should be people who can attest to your motivation, drive, and suitability for a career in medicine.

Selecting the wrong letter writers can really hurt your application. The best letters of recommendation are those that are submitted from a pre-health committee. They should include individual letters or excerpts from faculty, supervisors, and other people who know you well. If your college or university does not have a pre-health committee, letters of recommendation from faculty may be acceptable, but please be sure you ask faculty members who know you well.

Check with each medical school regarding the specific letters they require. Be sure that all your letters of recommendation are submitted on letterhead. If they are not, then they may not be acceptable. It is also important that your entire name, including middle name and AAMC ID, be listed on each letter submitted, to avoid confusion with another applicant who may have the same or a similar name. You can also help to avoid such confusion by reminding your letter writers to use your full name in their letters of recommendation.

Interfolio
www.interfolio.com

Applicants use Interfolio as an online tool to store, manage, and deliver their letters of recommendation to approximately seventy medical schools. Applicants can create an online portfolio at Interfolio and track their letters of recommendation. This makes things much easier for the letter writer, the medical schools, and the applicant.

VirtualEvals
www.virtualevals.org

This electronic service was designed to enhance the efficiency of how letters of recommendation are sent to the admissions offices at medical schools. Letters of recommendation are transmitted electronically from your undergraduate college or university to the admissions offices of the colleges to which you are applying. This has allowed the letter of recommendation process to become much more efficient and cost effective.

Applicants do not have access to VirtualEvals. Only the senders and receivers of the letters have access, so it is a very secure and confidential way to send letters of recommendation.

Check out their Web site to see what VirtualEvals is all about, what the advantages are, which medical schools participate, which undergraduate schools participate, and how it all started.

AMCAS Letter of Recommendation Service
www.aamc.org/students/amcas/faq/amcasletters.htm

Take advantage of the new letter writer service offered by AMCAS. This service allows medical schools the opportunity to receive all your letters of recommendation electronically via AMCAS. This will make things much easier for your letter writers, as it will allow them the opportunity just to send your letters directly to AMCAS, which will then send them electronically to each of the participating schools that you designate. According to AMCAS, 116 medical schools participate in this service for the fall 2010 application cycle.

Many undergraduate colleges and universities are now using VirtualEvals, Interfolio, or the AMCAS online letter of recommendation services to transmit applicants' letters of recommendation to the various medical schools. This is one of the best ways for a medical school to receive your letters of recommendation. This method ensures that they will not be lost in the mail, that they can be downloaded by the medical schools with ease, and that applicants can also confirm that they have been received by each medical school.

Check to see whether your school uses VirtualEvals, Interfolio, or the AMCAS service and whether the medical schools to which you are applying accept letters of recommendation via these services.

33. Be sure that your letter writers know you on a personal level.

It is difficult for admissions staff to evaluate letters written by people who do not know the student well. It is not helpful when your letter says, "Jane Doe was a student in my introduction to biology course. She was in the top 10% of her class of 300 students. She did well academically, earning a solid 'A' in my course. I think she will be successful in medical school and eventually make a great doctor." A form letter from a distinguished department chair will do more harm than a personal letter from a mere instructor who knows your academic capabilities and your character and is willing to write specifically about you.

It is important that your recommender says something about you that is not obvious in your application. She or he should discuss what kind of person you are, what kind of student you have been, what you have been able to offer your classmates, and the contributions you have made to class discussions, as well as commenting on your character, integrity, drive, and motivation. Therefore, it is imperative that these letters be written by and requested of people who have a solid familiarity with you and your desire to enter medical school and pursue a career as a physician.

34. Limit the number of letters of recommendation that you submit.

Every medical school has different requirements, so know what they are. Some schools will not accept more than two letters of recommendation, while others will only accept letters from faculty in particular disciplines, and others may only accept a letter from a health professions committee. If you submit fifteen letters of recommendation to a particular medical school, they will not all be read. Admissions committees will select the letters that they think are the most relevant.

If you wish to submit an additional or supplemental letter or two, contact the school to see if this is acceptable. An additional letter from a science faculty member or a supplemental letter from someone who has observed you volunteering with patients and can comment on how you came early, stayed late, easily established rapport with patients and doctors, and asked relevant questions may help your candidacy.

35. Make sure that your letters of recommendation are relevant.

Do not submit a letter of recommendation from the physician who fixed your broken arm when you were five. Applicants often make this mistake. They think that an M.D. after a recommender's name will greatly influence their chances of acceptance. If the letter writer does not know you well, the letter will not mean much to the admissions committee. Be thoughtful and selective in asking people to write your letters of recommendation.

36. Do not have your parents write a letter of recommendation.

Yes, it really happens — and probably more often than you would think! Of course, your parents are going to say how wonderful you are; they love you! Admissions committees are looking for letters that describe many different characteristics about you. They are looking for far more than what your parents can offer.

37. Do not write your own letters of recommendation and forge someone else's signature.

This seems obvious, but it has been attempted several times. It is very likely that the admissions committee will detect the fraud and then your chances of going to medical school will be gone forever!

Falsifying any part of your application will lead to the automatic rejection of your application. Don't even try it; it is not worth it!

38. Waive your rights to access your letters of recommendation.

It is in your best interest to waive your rights to your letters of recommendation. If you refuse, admissions committee members may wonder if there is something that you are trying to hide. It also casts doubt on whether your letter writers will be completely open in their assessment of you if you will have access to their letters. Some pre-med advisors, in fact, will not submit a letter of recommendation on the student's behalf if the student has not waived his or her rights.

The Personal Statement

The personal statement or essay is probably one of the most important parts of the application. It really is the only place in the screening process that you actually become a living, breathing person! You need to make yourself stand out and make the reader want to get to know more about you. This is a great place to tell your story. Who are you? What are you all about? How did you get to this point? Was there a particular experience that led you to the field of medicine? Was there a particular patient or physician that made you realize that pursuing a career in medicine was the right move for you?

Polish your essay in every way possible! Make sure it flows, is written well, and tells the reader exactly what you want it to say about you. Have someone who does not know you well read it. Do they get a true sense of who you are and why you are pursuing a medical career?

Do not reiterate everything in your application when writing your personal statement. There is no need to talk about your MCAT scores, your GPA, or where you went to undergraduate school. Write about something that makes you special and may set you apart from the other applicants.

Be careful that relevant experiences or activities are not hidden in your personal statement. List these experiences in the experiences section and discuss specifics about them in your personal statement. Sometimes students discuss their clinical experiences in the personal statement only, and the significance and specifics of these experiences get lost.

39. Do not quote Robert Frost in your personal statement.

Be original. Quotes from Robert Frost are very popular on medical school applications. You should probably leave him out of the process. You can be serious or use a bit of humor, but be creative, original, and yourself.

One student, with research experience in entomology, began his essay by comparing the different roles of ants in an ant colony to the role of a health professional. By the end of the essay, not only had he built a convincing point for the similarities, but his creative approach had also made his application stand out among the other applications.

Another non-traditional applicant began by stating how his responsibilities as a reference librarian for the past eleven years were similar to the responsibilities of a physician. Again, this made the reader pause to ask, "What similarities could possibly exist between these two very different positions?" By the end of the essay he had demonstrated, using humor and creativity, that his experiences had helped him to develop the strengths necessary to become a dedicated medical student and eventually a physician. At the same time, he was able to convey all the reasons why he was applying to medical school as a non-traditional student and what it was about him that made him special.

The Personal Statement in a Nutshell

Format:
  Short separated paragraphs.
  Perfect grammar.
  Avoid creative or unconventional formatting
    (screenplay, poems).
Content:
  Write it for your best friend.
Read it out loud:
  Is it clear?
Avoid puffery, name dropping, inauthentic quotes.
Tell a story.
Be honest but avoid confusion.

40. Use spellcheck and proofread your entire application.

Spellcheck will not pick up words used incorrectly, poor grammar, or run-on sentences. Proofread your personal statement very carefully. Read your essay, reread your essay, then reread your essay again. Does it make sense to you? Allow some time to lapse between readings. If you read your essay twelve times in the same day obvious errors may be easily missed. Let a day or two pass, then revisit your essay again. This will allow you to look at it with a fresh perspective.

Then have someone else read your personal statement, preferably someone who does not know you very well. Does it make sense to him or her? Does he or she get a good sense of who you are and the message that you are trying to convey? Keep in mind that this is the only part of the application where you really have the opportunity to individualize yourself outside your numbers. Will the reader be left with a strong impression of who you are, what you are all about, and your suitability for a career in medicine?

41. If you are applying to medical school and you want to be a physician, be sure to spell "physician" correctly.

"Physician," "pediatrician," "orthopedic surgeon" ... If you want to be one, be sure you know how to spell it! You would be surprised at how often this occurs and how many applications end up in the "no thank you" pile as a result of such carelessness.

42. When putting together your personal statement, do not generalize or criticize all doctors.

Do not forget that physicians will be reviewing your application; therefore it is probably not a good strategy to suggest that most physicians are incompetent and you are going to be the ideal doctor and will rescue our health care system. Also, be mindful of the fact that the people evaluating your application have many different backgrounds and credentials. For example, do not insult D.O. programs, as a D.O. may be one of your interviewers or sit on the committee deciding on your application.

Gimme a Break!

If you are considering any of the following, you might want to reconsider your personal statement!

"The possibility that I might discover a drug that could revolutionize medicine, coupled with my love for learning, is why I have chosen to pursue research this semester."

"I was able to overcome this mentally and emotionally stressful point in my life due to my undeterred and undying passion for a career in medicine."

"While volunteering at my local hospital, I often had a gut-wrenching feeling of helplessness."

"Suddenly I heard the crunch of metal against bone, and blood spattered everywhere. Everyone lost their heads in the ensuing moments except me. Thanks to my cool-headed actions, we were able to get our neighbor's dog to the vet in time."

43. Be careful not to start every sentence in your essay or personal statement with "I."

Admissions committees want to learn about you, but be careful that it does not sound like bragging. There is a fine line between confidence and overconfidence or cockiness. A narrative about some experience you have had might make your application stand out, but be careful not to inflate the importance of what you have done. Be honest as well as modest.

44. Keep your essay clear and well organized.

An essay with no breaks or paragraphs is hard to read, especially when yours might be one among several hundred that an admissions officer might be reading or reviewing in an afternoon. Always be conscious of how things will look to the person who is evaluating your application. If your essay is difficult to read or poorly organized, it may get overlooked.

45. Watch colloquialisms and profanity in your personal statement.

Admissions committees actually do read personal statements. They are a really important aspect of an application. Quoting a profanity in a pertinent personal story can be risky. What seems to you to be a vivid recreation could actually offend some members of the admissions committee. Why take that chance?

You know the words to avoid, but do not forget the more common slang words that do not sound very professional: "sucks," "bastard," "dude," "awesome," and so on.

Experiences — Clinical, Research, Volunteer, and Extracurricular Activities

It is important that you choose your activities carefully. Not only are admissions committees looking for academically qualified students, but they are also looking for students who are self-motivated and dedicated to serving others. They are seeking compassionate, caring, and honest students who possess high ethical standards and can effectively manage their time.

By getting involved in a variety of different experiences you are showing the admissions committee that you are well-rounded and able to handle multiple activities at once, all the while maintaining a solid academic performance. It is important to show the admissions committee that you can successfully balance your school work with all your outside activities. This will help them to evaluate your ability to handle the demands of your life as a physician. Most medical schools are looking for a combination of clinical experiences in which you shadow physicians and have patient contact, extracurricular activities and leadership opportunities, community service or volunteer work, and research experiences.

What About Those Extracurricular Activities?

Name the activity, your role in it, and the depth of your involvement.
Prefer few but intense rather than many "boutique" contacts.
Emphasize direct patient contact.
Cite non-medical service as well.
Catalogue them honestly.

46. Do not try to impress the admissions committee with everything you have ever done in your entire life.

Things that you did during junior high are probably not relevant to anything at this level. If you want the admissions committee to know of your longstanding interest in being a physician, your personal statement is probably the best place for this.

47. Adequately describe each activity and experience.

Do not simply list your activities like you would on a resumé. Use complete sentences and punctuation, elaborate on your experiences, and make clear to the reader how each activity might be relevant to your success in medical school. Do not leave out pertinent information regarding each of your experiences for the sake of brevity. Be concise, but also highlight your responsibilities and what you got out of each experience.

While you should not try to use every character space that AMCAS allots you to describe each experience, do not miss the opportunity to describe and "sell" each experience. For example, if you have research experience, describe your research and your role or responsibilities. If perhaps you suggested a new approach that was implemented or were given more responsibility, mention this! Perhaps you volunteered in the emergency room, where your primary role was to interview and transport patients, but on occasion were given the opportunity to go on rounds or observe an interesting procedure or case. Mention this!

48. Be careful not to "pad" your resumé with things you think the committee wants to see.

Be careful that you are not selecting activities just because you think they will look good on your medical school application. Leadership roles are very important. Spend a significant amount of time doing things that you enjoy — and do them well. Admissions committees are looking for quality over quantity. Find a balance that you are comfortable with and that combines academics, extracurricular activities, work, and family. No one wants you to give up your entire life to prepare for your medical school application, so continue doing the things that are important to you.

49. Remember, there are only 168 hours in a week.

Be sure, when you are adding up your school work, class time, extracurricular activities, shadowing, and research experiences, that they do not add up to more than 168 hours. Be realistic, truthful, and accurate when filling out your activities page. If you have a lot of activities and your grades have suffered as a result of overextending yourself, this will not work in your favor.

50. Being a bridesmaid is not an extracurricular activity and giving blood once a year is not a volunteer activity ...

... and surfing the Web is not a hobby. Be careful about the impression that activities like this will make on members of the admissions committee. They are looking for substantial, quality experiences that tell them something about who you are and the things that you are passionate about. The activities that you list should reflect your interests and serve as a possible indicator of how committed you are to service work, how well you work with others, and how well you manage your time.

If you consider giving blood once a year a volunteer activity, then you had better get out there and get some additional volunteer experiences. Although this is a good start, it really does not say enough about your dedication to serving others and your drive to be a physician. It is viewed as "the right thing to do," but is not going to be enough to prove your dedication to serving others.

51. Timing is essential.

It is important that your experiences and activities be an ongoing process. Do not start your extracurricular experiences right before applying to medical school. This will be viewed as simply getting the experiences because you have to, instead of doing them because of your own interest or desire.

Also, keep in mind that the applicant pool is filled with thousands of other highly qualified applicants, many of whom have known from an early stage that they wanted to become doctors, and who have a considerable amount of relevant activities. These are the people with whom you are going to be compared and against whom you will be competing for a limited number of seats.

> ### *What Should Your Activities Convey?*
>
> *I like to serve people. I can do this day after day.*
> *I have given medicine a good try, and I think I understand its*
> *joys and trials.*

52. Clinical experience is absolutely necessary.

You need to show the admissions committee that you have investigated the field of medicine and are sure that you know exactly what you are getting yourself into. It is important that you have a clear understanding of what physicians do during the day and how they interact with their patients, the families of their patients, and other health care professionals.

If you indicate that you are leaning toward a certain specialty, for example, pediatric orthopedic surgery, be prepared to discuss what you know about this specialty during your interview. Be able to discuss what you have observed, the day-to-day responsibilities of a pediatric orthopedic surgeon, the types of patients they usually see, and why you think you might enjoy this specialty area.

If you always thought you might enjoy being an oncologist or an otolaryngologist, then shadow physicians in these areas, in addition to those in other areas, to experience a variety of roles and responsibilities. This exploration will not only help you decide that medicine is the right career for you, but it will also help you to convey better in your personal statement or interview your reasons for wanting to enter the medical profession.

If you happen to be the child of a physician, it is important that you get additional clinical experiences shadowing other physicians and getting direct patient contact. This will show the admissions committee that this is something that **you** want and have investigated on your own, not simply something that you have heard your parent discuss at the dinner table.

Think of it like this: If an admissions officer has ten applications on the desk that all have about the same GPA and MCAT scores, but there is only one interview spot left, who will get this last interview spot? Most likely, the officer will offer it to the applicant with the most clinical experience, because that speaks volumes about how motivated he or she is, and about the fact that this candidate has already gotten a good amount of relevant experience. This edge may persuade the admissions officer to believe that this applicant probably has a realistic expectation of what he or she is about to take on. While perfect MCATs and a high GPA might reflect well on your aptitude for succeeding academically in medical school, they do not reveal anything specific about your motivation for or your understanding of the medical profession. Clinical experience often does.

53. Continuing clinical experience is a must.

It is incredibly important for you to continue any relevant clinical experience. Having good quality, ongoing experience will show your genuine motivation for medicine. Just because you already have done several summers of volunteer work does not mean that you should stop now. You really should continue to be involved throughout your senior year and the entire application cycle.

54. Tell the truth!

Everything in your application is "fair game." If you listed it, be prepared to talk about it during an interview. Admissions committee members have been known to call the "contact person" whom you list in your experiences. Be sure that you have done what you say you have done. If you are in the process of founding an organization, say that. Do not say you already founded it, only to have a member of the admissions committee check with your undergraduate college and find that the organization does not yet exist.

55. Volunteer work is very important.

Countless students have said that they are interested in the field of medicine because they want to help people. If this is why you are going into medicine, be sure that your application contains evidence that you have helped people. Being a physician means that you will be dedicating your life to serving others. You need to be sure you want this.

One way to convey your commitment to service work is by volunteering and trying to make a difference in your community. Volunteer for Hospice, become a literacy volunteer or a Big Brother or Big Sister. Get out there, get involved, and make a difference!

56. Research experiences are not required at every medical school, so investigate which schools require or recommend research.

Some schools do require research. They think that it is a very important part of the medical profession and is the foundation for medical knowledge. Over the course of your career, you will need to utilize various forms of medical literature to treat your future patients and remain current in your field.

It is important for you to apply to schools that are consistent with your own interest, or lack of interest, in research. Do not do research just because you think you have to; do it because you really want to do it.

If you have done research, be prepared to talk about it. You will need to be able to describe your project in detail and discuss exactly what role you played in the research.

If you are unable to describe or explain your research, your duties, or your findings, then the admissions committee will be left wondering if this is a case of embellishment. If you have simply done research for the sake of having it look good on a medical school application, this will be easily detected.

You also may want to explore non-scientific research as well. This could be a great opportunity to show independent thinking, an appreciation for the process of research, and a slant toward lifelong learning without being limited to working with pipettes!

The Interview Process

You got the call, and you have a medical school interview. Now what? The interview can truly make or break your candidacy. The committee saw something that they liked in your application. They want to learn more about you, to find out what you have to offer the field of medicine, and to see if their medical school is the right fit for you.

Be kind, courteous, respectful, and professional to everyone you come into contact with. Prepare for your interviews and do your homework on each medical school. Practice your interviews — but not to the point where your answers sound rehearsed. Prepare questions to ask your interviewers, review your AMCAS application, and keep in mind that you are evaluating the medical schools just as much as they are evaluating you.

While most applicants focus on the fact that they are going to be evaluated during their interviews, many are unaware that schools view the interview not just as a means of evaluating them as candidates, but also as a marketing tool. Scheduling and conducting interviews requires a lot of effort. If you have been invited for an interview, it is because a school has seen something in your application that made them want to meet you in person to learn more about you. Medical schools want to make good impressions on the competitive applicants whom they invite to campus, showing off their newest facilities, their happy students, and their distinguished faculty. They want competitive applicants to leave their campus impressed with all they have to offer and wanting to attend!

If you are traveling a long distance for several interviews, it is acceptable to contact the admissions offices at the schools to let them know you will be in the area during a particular time and would be happy to come in for an interview. If the school will be granting you an interview, they may be able to grant your request, saving you time and money.

> ### *The Medical School Interview*
>
> *Have some explanations, but do not overpractice.*
> *Do not criticize; do not make excuses.*
> *Do not be drawn into being an expert ... if you are not.*
> *This is not confession.*

57. It is not necessary to wear a black suit, white shirt, and red tie.

It is important to dress professionally, but spice it up a bit and be a little different. With that said, be careful not to be too casual or too revealing in your attire. Women should wear a pantsuit or skirt and blouse. Men should wear a suit or khakis and sports jacket with a shirt and tie.

58. Get enough sleep and be well rested for your interview.

It is important to be at your best during your interview. Applicants have actually fallen asleep during group interviews and then awakened to ask a question that had already been covered. If necessary, get up, walk out, and compose yourself, rather than embarrassing yourself by nodding off.

59. Do not go out and get "smashed" the night before your interview.

If you happen to have friends in the vicinity of your interview and if you get together the night before your interview, try to keep it low key. If you do go out for a night on the town, be sure not to talk about the previous night's events in great detail with your interviewer or within earshot of the admissions director or a member of the admissions staff.

60. If your interviewer says something inappropriate or creates an uncomfortable interview situation for you, tell the admissions director.

If you do not tell the admissions director, he or she will never know that an interviewer is not behaving appropriately. It is important that you speak up before a decision has been made on your application, as decisions are often final. After you have been waitlisted or rejected, your concerns may seem less valid. Let the admissions director know about your concerns prior to leaving on interview day. Once you leave, there may not be anything that can be done to help you or to rectify the situation.

Possible Questions to Ask
During Your Interview

Please describe the medical school curriculum. (Is it problem-based? Organ-based?)

Are the lectures taped?

Is there a note-taking service?

Is a PDA or laptop required?

Can you tell me about the international opportunities available? (Summers and electives?)

Is there patient contact in the first year?

Can you tell me about the research opportunities for students?

What is the grading system like? (Pass/fail? Modified A/B/C?)

Is this a very competitive environment?

Are there support services available? (Personal counseling, tutoring, advising?)

Are the match statistics available?

May I send updated materials for the admissions committee to consider?

Are there any special programs that this medical school is known for?

How do students perform on the boards?

How accessible are the faculty?

How are students evaluated during their clinical years?

Are there extracurricular activities available?

Is a car necessary for clinical rotations?

Are students allowed to participate on medical school committees?

Are students involved in community service projects, either required or voluntary?

What made you choose to complete your medical education here?

What made you decide to work here?

What do you think the school's greatest strengths are?

What do you see changing here over the next four years?

61. Always come to your interview prepared with questions for your interviewers.

If you have two interviewers and the first one answered your questions, ask again; another perspective is always helpful. If you have no questions, you could be viewed as being uninterested in the institution. Medical schools want to accept applicants who want to be there and are enthusiastic about their program and institution.

This is your opportunity to learn more about the medical school in order to help you decide whether or not it is the right "fit" for you. Can you see yourself there? Would you be happy there if accepted? Does the school offer the social and academic experiences that you are looking for in your medical education? If you are curious about clinical experiences, the curriculum, or what type of academic support services they offer to students, this is the perfect opportunity to find out more!

Do not, however, pepper your interviewers with questions that could easily be answered by viewing the school's Web site or from the materials that you have received. Your questions need to be genuine and should come naturally out of the conversation.

62. Do not try to be someone that you are not.

Most experienced interviewers can detect an insincere applicant. Interviews are designed to get to know who you are and to see if this particular medical school is the right medical school for you. Relax and be yourself.

63. If you are running late for your interview, be sure to call.

If you are caught in traffic, lost, or have missed a flight, be sure to call the admissions office right away and let them know. Most interview days are carefully planned and schedules can be pretty tight. There may not be a lot of wiggle room. Make sure to apologize if you are late so that the staff knows that you are taking this interview seriously.

Sometimes students become lax about their responsibilities when they already have an acceptance but are still interviewing. If you are really not interested in being there, cancel your interview as early as humanly possible. There are many other students who would be happy to take your interview spot.

64. Dress for the weather.

Do some homework on the climate where you will be interviewing. For instance, when applicants are interviewing in the month of January in Central New York, chances are that they will need coats, hats, gloves, boots, or umbrellas.

You never know how far you may have to walk for your interviews, campus tour, or parking. You do not want to show up at your interview late, wet, and shivering because you just trudged up a slush-covered hill in a skirt and dress shoes.

65. Turn off your cell phones.

If you must leave your cell phone on, put it on vibrate. You do not want some kind of funky ring tone like Kanye West's "Gold

Digger," Beyonce's "Irreplaceable," or Justin Timberlake's "SexyBack," going off during your interview. That would be embarrassing and inappropriate.

66. If you do keep your phone on, be polite.

Use common sense and good phone etiquette. If you **must** answer your phone while in the presence of an admissions staff member, do not hold up your finger indicating that you will only be a minute and that she or he should wait for you so that you can take the call — yes, this has really happened! Tell your caller that you will return the call as soon as possible, and apologize to the person whom you have just left waiting. Remember, everything that you do in the interview process reflects on how you might treat a patient or colleague.

67. Be prepared to talk about your institutional action(s), misdemeanors, felonies, etc.

The admissions committee will want to know as much as they can about any institutional actions or charges against you. Alcohol offenses, plagiarism, and academic probation seem to be the most common institutional violations. Plagiarism offenses and alcohol violations have become more common over the past few years. All such actions are serious and need to be addressed with candor and sincerity in your application. Several similar violations may be seen as a cause for concern and may affect how strongly your application is considered. Anticipate these areas of concern regarding your prior action(s) and think about how you are going to explain and account for your actions in the best possible light. Remember to be honest and frank in your explanation.

68. Be prepared to talk about pass/fail courses, withdrawing from courses, or repeating courses.

Interviews are the perfect opportunity for the admissions committee to get answers to questions that they have about your academic past. They are looking for clarification of any "red flags" that they see in your academic record. Be honest. Avoid blaming anyone, especially your professors. Focus on the positive, for example, what you have learned from the experience and how you have applied what you learned to ensure success in your future studies.

Be very careful in your explanations. Perhaps you withdrew from organic chemistry because you were taking a heavy course load and wanted to take it when you had a lighter schedule, and perhaps increase your chances of earning an "A." This may indicate to an interviewer that you are not up for the challenge of the medical school curriculum. It is also not a good idea to say you dropped a class because the professor was difficult and you wanted to take it the next semester with an "easier" professor.

69. Do not give "canned" answers to interview questions.

Although it is important to practice your interviews, interviewers are looking for genuine, unforced answers to their questions. You do not want to sound rehearsed — and please, do not answer their questions with answers that you think they want to hear, instead of what you really think or feel.

There might not always be a right or wrong answer to a question posed during an interview. The interview has more to do with how you express yourself than with what you say or know. Sometimes an applicant may give an answer to a question that he or she **wanted** the interviewer to ask rather than answering the question that was actually asked. This may call the applicant's listening skills into question. Ask for clarification if you do not understand the question.

Be sure to review your answers to your primary application as well as to the medical school's secondary application as part of your interview preparation. If you are asked a question about something you wrote about in your application and you respond with, "I am not sure what you are talking about. Could I please see the essay?" you will sound completely unprepared for your interview and will bring all the answers to the questions in your application into question.

70. Practice your interviews.

Try doing some mock interviews with someone at your career center or with someone you do not know very well. It will be very important that you do these in a setting similar to that in which you will be interviewing. Wear a suit, shake hands, sit across from your interviewer, have your interviewer prepare questions similar to those that may be asked. You will want to make this scenario as realistic as possible — and a little uncomfortable for you.

It is important that you interview well, but it is equally important not to sound rehearsed. If you do not know the answer to a particular question, it is okay to say that you do not know, but do your best to answer the question. The interviewer may not be looking for the "right" answer, but may instead be interested in seeing how you handle yourself or how you think.

You need to be able to answer basic questions. For instance, if you are asked what your three greatest strengths are, you need three, not two. You can find examples of frequently asked medical school interview questions online. You can also visit <www.studentdoctor.net> to view questions that other applicants were asked during their interviews. This preparation will help you to anticipate some of the questions that you may be asked.

Possible Interview Questions

Tell me about yourself.
What do you do in your spare time?
How would your friends describe you?
How did you select your undergraduate institution?
How did you select your major?
What undergraduate science class was your favorite and why?
What kinds of non-science courses have you taken, and how will you apply your experiences in those classes to a career in medicine?
What are your strengths (both academically and personally)?
What exposure have you had to the medical field?
Why do you want to be a doctor?
What have you done to solidify that medicine is the right career for you?
What makes you think you would be a good doctor?
Describe your research/clinical/volunteer experiences in medicine.
What are you looking for in a medical school?
What is it specifically about our medical school that made you want to apply?
What will you do if you are not accepted to medical school?
If you were not accepted to medical school, what other profession would you pursue?

71. Do not answer your interviewer's questions with one-word answers.

Often applicants are nervous about the interviews. It is okay to be nervous and even to admit that you are nervous, but be careful that your anxiety does not get the best of you. The interview is your chance to really "sell" yourself. Answering your interview questions with one-word answers will not allow your interviewer to get to know you very well. You **must** elaborate on your answers. The admissions committee wants to know as much as they can about you, and this may be your and their only opportunity for that.

It is important for you to demonstrate clearly your ability to articulate your thoughts and to communicate effectively. Effective communication skills are crucial when working with patients, their families, and as part of a team with other health professionals.

More Possible Interview Questions

If accepted to medical school, what do you think will be the greatest challenge in completing it?
How would you contribute to the student body here?
What sets you apart from other applicants?
How would you deal with another medical professional who holds differing views from yours?
What do you consider to be the biggest problem in health care today? How will you address it in your future career?
Where do you see yourself in ten years?
Why should we accept you?
What would you identify as weaknesses in your application?
What should I tell the admissions committee about you?
What personal accomplishment are you most proud of?
Who is your role model and why? How has that person inspired you to be who you are today?
Do you have any questions for me?

72. Send a thank-you note to your interviewers.

If you really enjoyed your interview experience, send a thank-you note to your interviewer(s) or student host. A personal handwritten card, a typed letter, or an e-mail are all acceptable ways to convey your appreciation.

Sometimes applicants are in such a rush to send these out that they might send one to the wrong school or the wrong person. If you do send thank-you notes, be sure that you send each one to the right person at the right medical school.

73. Do not tell your interviewers that their school is not your first choice.

You may think that this is obvious, and it really should be, but it happens more often than you would believe. During your interview, you must be able to say something special about a particular program or the school and what it was that made you want to apply there.

Take a brief moment to look over the curriculum or special programs offered, and find something specific that appeals to you and your interests. You will be better able to convey interest in a program (even if it is not your top choice) if you have taken some time to research the program to which you are applying.

With a limited number of seats available, why would a school want to award a seat to anyone who does not really want to be there? Why would you want to waste your time or money interviewing somewhere that you are really not interested in attending?

74. Answer honestly if an interviewer asks where else you have interviewed.

Try not to get defensive or paranoid if you are asked this question. Many times the interviewers are just curious to see which other medical schools you are considering. It will not be used against you. You do not necessarily have to name the names of the other schools. Instead, talk about the qualities that you find most attractive in a medical school. This gives the interviewer a sense of what you are looking for in a medical school — and why.

75. Do not bring your parents or significant other with you to your interview.

So you are thinking, "No kidding!" I wish I could say that it never happens, but it does! Moms, dads, girlfriends, and boyfriends should all be left at home. The interview process should demonstrate your independence and maturity. You do not want to stand out among the other applicants and be remembered as the applicant who brought his or her mom along to the medical school interview. They are more than welcome to attend most "Second Look" or "Second Visit" days, if you really want them to see the medical schools that you are considering. But on interview day, their presence is just not appropriate.

76. Make the most of your interview day.

Sit in on classes, check out the library or the computer clusters, hang out in the student lounge, or take a walk outside to see what the local community is like.

Sitting in on classes is critically important. Not only will you learn how the classes are taught, but you can observe the dynamics between the faculty and the students and among the students themselves. How do the students interact with one another and with their professors? Does the environment appear to be cutthroat or supercompetitive?
Is the faculty interested in the material they are presenting? Do they seem approachable? Do class interactions fit with the environment for which you are looking? Do the students appear to be happy?

Your day on campus is your best opportunity to determine whether or not this medical school is the right fit for you.

77. Ask current students about their experiences.

See if you can spend the night before your interview with a current student; he or she is your best resource! Not only can this save you money, but it is also a great way to learn more about a particular medical school. Contact the admissions office in advance. They often can put you in touch with students who have volunteered to host applicants the night before their interviews.

Whenever you have the opportunity, talk to current students about their own experiences. They have been where you are and know what you are going through, and they are often happy to share their personal experiences with prospective students.

Questions To Ask Current Students

What do they like about the medical school?
Are there things they do not like?
Why did they choose this particular medical school?
Is it competitive or cutthroat?
Are they happy here?
What makes the school stand out?
How accessible is the faculty?
Are there any special programs?
What is the town or city like?
What have their clinical experiences been like?
When did they first have patient contact?
What is the curriculum like?
Are they happy with the curriculum?
What kind of residency planning is available?
*Is there counseling, tutoring, and other assistance
        available?*
Do they recommend the support services?

78. You are always "on the record."

Keep in mind that there is always some type of evaluation process taking place, even if it is informal or "off the record." Always be polite and respectful.

If student hosts take you in and allow you to stay overnight in their home, be thankful. Sometimes they are studying for exams, and they are always busy. Do not cast aspersions toward them by insulting their school, the school to which you are applying, while you are staying with them.

When applying to a medical school, you are **asking** them to honor your request for admission. It is important to keep in mind that entry into medical school is a **privilege** and not a right, no matter how outstanding an applicant's grades or experiences are.

79. Bring a book or something to do during down time.

Chances are there will be a bit of down time during your interview day, so be prepared to wait. For some of you it will be too much time; for others of you it will not be enough. Making everyone happy is difficult. Bring a book along so you can catch up on some pleasure reading. If you are asked the question, "What is the last book you read?" you will then be able to provide a quick answer.

Take advantage of this opportunity. This may also be a great time to do some of the things mentioned previously: sit in on classes, look over the campus, go to the library, grab a coffee in the cafeteria, visit the student lounge, etc. Use this time to learn more about whether or not you can realistically see yourself as happy at this medical school.

80. Watch how you shake hands.

Be confident and look your interviewer in the eye. A good, strong handshake is incredibly important. There is nothing worse than a sweaty or especially a limp handshake, which may showcase a passive or insecure demeanor.

81. Be sure to bring extra cash on your interview day.

Always plan on a little more money than you think you might need for incidentals. You may be surprised at the cost of parking, taxis, porters, and food. You also should not assume that you can use a debit or credit card. It may be embarrassing to have to borrow money from the director of admissions to get your car out of the parking garage.

82. Eat breakfast.

Catch the continental breakfast at your hotel on your interview day. Most medical schools do not serve breakfast, and it may be a while before you are served lunch. Eating breakfast will also help you to wake up and have a clear mind for your interviews.

83. Do not complain about the lunch you are served at your interview.

If you have specific restrictions (e.g., kosher, vegetarian, etc.), then be sure to notify the medical school at least one week prior to your interview day. Many schools have their lunches catered and must place their orders several days in advance.

84. Do not be too casual during your interview.

Some interviewers take a formal approach to interviewing, while others might prefer to be more conversational in their approach. Even if an interviewer takes a more laid back approach, remember that you are **still** being interviewed and that you are applying to a professional school. Do not lean back in your chair and put your feet up on the table or be too cavalier in your responses. Interviewers do not want to hear about how you like to "chill" in your free time and "kick it" with your friends.

85. When asked about end-of-life issues, respond with appropriate dignity.

Although end-of-life issues may make you uncomfortable, be thoughtful with your responses. Please do not say, "I don't have a problem with dead people," or, "It's good to tell jokes to lighten the mood."

Death is an issue that you will no doubt have to confront as a physician. How will you handle losing a patient? Are you comfortable with death? What experience, if any, do you have with death? How do you feel about a patient's right to die? Or euthanasia? Reflect on these questions and know where you stand on these topics. You may be asked some tough ethical questions during your interview, so be prepared.

86. Be prepared for interview day surprises.

Ask questions about the different interview days at each medical school before your interviews. Talk to your pre-health advisor and check out the medical school Web site, or take a look at the interview feedback section at <www.studentdoctor.net>.

Talk to other students who have interviewed where you are interviewing. It is important to know how the interviews are structured and conducted. Will there be stress interviews, surprise essays, panel interviews, student interviewers? Which components of your application will each of your interviewers have? Will it be a closed file interview, where your interviewer does not have any information about you other than your name? Knowing this information ahead of time may make your interview day much less stressful.

87. If you can, find out in advance who will be interviewing you.

You may not know who is interviewing you until the morning you arrive on campus. If a computer is available and if you can find out who will be interviewing you, you can use some of your down time to learn about your interviewer on the college Web site. Your extra effort in this regard could make you stand out and might also reveal some common interests between you and your interviewer.

88. Try to relax enough to be interested in your interviewer.

This may help you to reduce your anxiety. Who is this person? What does he or she do? How does she or he view the institution? How long has he or she been here? How can her or his experience shed light on the institution and on your understanding about whether it might be a good fit for you?

Your ability to demonstrate interest in your interviewer could be seen as a surrogate for the interest that you will eventually have in your patients. The ability to meet a stranger and engage in an open, mutually satisfying dialogue demonstrates good potential for doctoring, a profession where you will need to meet strangers and establish rapport quickly on a daily basis.

89. Do not panic if your interviewer does not ask every question there is to ask about you.

Interviews are mostly designed to recruit students. If you feel that something very relevant to your candidacy was overlooked, or if you want to add something that was not covered in your interview, it may be appropriate to submit a follow-up letter to the admissions committee. At the end of your interview, you may also ask your interviewer to share a particular piece of information with the admissions committee.

Overall, let the interviewer control the interview and the flow of conversation. Perhaps your interviewer loves opera and you are an accomplished singer. It is okay if the interview centers around that interest. Most interviewers are trying to gain a sense of your overall maturity, intelligence, compassion, and depth. An experienced interviewer can assess all these things by asking questions that are not medically related.

90. If you have the opportunity to interview with a current student, do it!

Current students can offer you some really great insight into the college and into medical school life. They have been through this challenging process and are now living the lives of medical students. They are often very willing to discuss their experiences, decisions, and even regrets, and to give you their honest opinions about the program they have chosen. Student interviewers are usually not paid, but volunteer their time to help the admissions office select the best applicants for the next year's entering class.

Student interviewers tend to look at prospective students very differently. They seem to assess students more as potential colleagues than as potential medical students. Chances are they may be working alongside you or referring patients to you one day.

91. Do not leave the interview day early.

Leaving before the campus tour or the end of your interview day sends a bad message about your level of interest in attending the medical school you are visiting. Medical schools are looking for not only the most qualified students, but also students who want to be there. It costs time and money to travel around the country and attend each interview for medical school, so why not relax and find out as much as you can about each school?

Be sure to plan your travel according to the interview schedule at the medical school. Do not show up the morning of your interview and tell the admissions staff that you need to leave by noon to catch a flight, when you have been told that you will need to remain on campus until at least 3:00. Making the admissions office scramble to accommodate your schedule is not the way you want to be remembered.

92. Be conscious of your non-verbal communication during the interview.

Look your interviewer in the eye. Eye contact, facial expressions, posture, and hand gestures are all incredibly important! It is also important to respect a person's personal space.

Top Five Non-Verbals
for Interviewing

According to <collegegrad.com>, many interviews fail because of lack of proper communication. But communication is more than just what you say. Often it is the non-verbal communication that we are least aware of, that speaks the loudest. Following are the top five non-verbals, ranked in order of importance, when it comes to interviewing:

Eye Contact — Unequaled in importance! If you have a habit of looking away while listening, it shows a lack of interest and a short attention span. If you fail to maintain eye contact while speaking, it might convey a lack of confidence or send a subtle indication that you might be lying. Don't just assume that you have good eye contact. Ask. Watch. Practice. Ask others if you ever lack proper eye contact. If so, was it during speaking or listening? Sit down with a friend and practice until you are comfortable maintaining sincere, continuous eye contact.

Facial Expressions — Take a good, long, hard look at yourself in the mirror. Look at yourself as others would. Do you look scared? Bored? Engaged? Add a simple feature that nearly every interviewee forgets – smile! A true and genuine smile says that you are a happy person and delighted to be interviewing today.

Posture — Posture sends signals of confidence. Stand tall, walk tall, and, most of all, sit tall. When you are seated, make sure that you sit at the front edge of the chair, slightly leaning forward, intent on the subject at hand.

Gestures — Gestures should be limited during the interview. Do not use artificial gestures to heighten the

> *importance of the issue at hand. You will merely come off as theatrical. When you do use gestures, make sure that they are sincere and meaningful.*
>
> *Space — Recognize the boundaries of your personal space and that of others. If you are typical of most Americans, it will range between 30 and 36 inches. Be prepared, however, not to back up or move away from someone who has a personal space that is smaller than your own. Hang in there, take a deep breath, and stand your ground. For most of us, being aware of our personal space is enough to prompt us to stand firm. If you have a smaller than average personal space, make sure you keep your distance so that you do not intimidate someone who needs more room.*

93. Be flexible! Try not to get too irritated if there is a last-minute change during your interview day.

A day in the life of any physician is unpredictable. You will often have to deal with less than perfect situations when patients or colleagues do inconvenient things at very inconvenient times. Do not complain! You need to be able to roll with these changes.

94. Do not tell your interviewer that you are going into medicine for prestige or money.

If that is why you want to be a doctor, then you should find a new profession. There are people who work much less and make much more money than physicians. You can make more money as an investment banker and usually incur less debt. A career in medicine will be a long, lonely, and hard road if you are in it for the wrong reasons!

Waiting for a Decision

It can seem to take forever when you are waiting for an admissions decision. Most medical schools cannot begin sending out admissions decisions until October 15. If you interview in early September, a month and a half is a long wait.

Be sure to ask the following questions during your interview day: How long until a decision is made? How will you hear from the admissions committee, by a status page on the school Web site, by phone call, e-mail, or postal mail? If you are put on a waitlist, how does the alternate list work? Are students reevaluated? Is the list ranked? Can you send in new information? If you are denied admission, is there advisement available? Often, your interviewer will not know the answers to these questions, but the admissions staff and director will certainly be able to help you.

95. Be patient!

Chances are that you will not hear from an admissions committee for four to six weeks, or even longer, after your interview. You are welcome to check in to see if a decision has been made on your application, but be careful not to call or e-mail too often.

96. Do not contact your interviewers to find out "what went wrong" if you are denied admission.

Sometimes medical school interviewers are not members of the medical school admissions committee, and while they do offer their recommendations to the committee, they may not be present or part of the actual voting process when the decision on your application is made. The committee looks at the big picture and takes everything into account — grades and MCAT scores, extracurricular activities, clinical exposure, research experience, work-related experience, letters of recommendation, interviewer ratings, and the overall competitiveness of the applicant pool that year. To find out how to strengthen your application, it is probably best to talk to your pre-health advisor or a member of the medical school admissions staff, if the school offers such advisement.

97. Take advantage of any "Second Visit Day" opportunities at the medical schools to which you have been accepted.

"Second Visit" or "Second Look" days are great opportunities to revisit the medical schools that you are truly interested in. This time you will be more seriously evaluating what each medical school has to offer you, what makes it unique, and whether it is the right fit for you. Since you are no longer being evaluated, this visit should be much more relaxed, and you can evaluate the school through different eyes. This visit may be a good time to bring your parents, spouse, or significant other to have them help you evaluate your options. Dress comfortably and leave your suit at home, but be sure to check to see if there is a particular dress code for different events that you might be attending.

Reapplying

Do not reapply unless you have spent adequate time making significant changes to your application. These changes usually come in the form of new grades, MCAT scores, experiences, different letters of recommendation, and a new personal statement. This will take a great deal of preparation and is not something that can be accomplished in just a short period of time.

First, go back and talk to your pre-health advisor to seek his or her advice about what you should do differently for your next round of applications. Second, while not all medical schools offer application counseling to applicants, if you have the opportunity to meet with an admissions person and go over your application, do it. They are the people reviewing your application and can best point out the strengths and weaknesses of your application. Do not assume that you know what the problem was with your application. It may be something entirely different than what you suspect.

If you were interviewed and later rejected, ask for **honest** feedback from the admissions staff at one or more of the medical schools that interviewed you. If you are able to speak to a member of the admissions staff, be open to their feedback and suggestions and do not become defensive. It is important that you take their comments seriously. If you received multiple interviews that resulted in waitlists or post-interview rejections, chances are that your interviews are your weak point and you should improve this skill before interviewing again.

98. Do not, under any circumstances, resubmit the same application.

Make positive changes to your application. If it did not work the first time, chances are that same application is not going to work the second time. Most medical schools will keep application records for a couple of years, and if an applicant resubmits exactly the same application, particularly the same personal statement or letters of recommendation, it will probably be rejected because there is nothing new to evaluate.

How motivated could someone be to become a physician if he or she could not even take the time to write a new personal statement or to request current letters of recommendation? The admissions staff wants to know what you have done to strengthen your application since last applying; they will be looking for changes and improvements in your qualifications. How has the past year or years served to increase your drive and motivation to become a physician?

99. If poor grades were the biggest problem with your previous application, do not reapply until you have nearly finished a postbaccalaureate or graduate program.

If you reapply as soon as you enter the program, there will not be enough time to show the admissions committee that you can handle a rigorous science curriculum or graduate-level coursework. Besides, it is unlikely that your grades will be available in time for the admissions committee to consider them. If it is a two-year program, you need to plan on completing the program. A condition of acceptance at many schools is that you successfully complete your current program of study. Do not enroll in any program from which you plan to withdraw if you are accepted to medical school.

In some cases, one semester of postbaccalaureate or graduate coursework may not be enough to overcome a previous poor academic record. It is best to relax, do well, and take some time to prove your academic ability and consistency to the admissions committee.

100. Do not assume that because you were on a school's waitlist or alternate list last year, you have a better chance of gaining acceptance this year.

Each year's applicant pool is different from the year before, and most schools will look at applicants independently from year to year. In addition, medical schools may be looking for different things each year when reviewing applications. Think of every application and every interview as a new opportunity to sell yourself to the medical school.

Alternate Lists

If you are placed on a medical school's alternate or waitlist, call to see if they will accept any additional information from you for further review of your application. You may want to touch base with the medical school to see how their list is moving and to let them know that you are still interested in attending, should an opening arise. Be sure that they have your correct contact information on file.

Many schools will not release much information regarding the movement of their alternate lists. They may tell you generic information, such as whether you are in the top third, middle third, or bottom third, but they may not tell you how many students are on their list. Some will keep an active alternate list up until the first day of orientation.

Most Importantly ...

101. Always, always be yourself!

Applying to medical school is a very long and often overwhelming process. Applicants can sometimes get caught up in the "They have to like me" or "I will do whatever it takes" attitude to gain acceptance to medical school. But it is very important that you always remain true to yourself, from your thoughts about pursuing a career in medicine, to your application, and to your interview.

Be the person you are, instead of the person you think the medical school is looking for. Every school is different, but you need to go where you feel most comfortable. Choose a school that is truly the right fit for you.

Web Sites

American Association of Colleges of Osteopathic
Medicine Application Service
<aacomas.aacom.org>

American Medical College Application Service
<www.aamc.org/amcas>

AMCAS Letters of Evaluation / Recommendation
<www.aamc.org/students/amcas/faq/amcasletters.htm>

AAMC FACTS <www.aamc.org/data/facts>

AAMC Background Check Service
<www.aamc.org/students/amcas/faq/background.htm>

AAMC Publications <www.aamc.org/publications>

CollegeGrad.com <www.collegegrad.com>

Free Application for Federal Student Aid (FAFSA)
<www.fafsa.ed.gov>

Interfolio <www.interfolio.com>

Medical College Admission Test (MCAT) <www.aamc.org/mcat>

National Association of Advisors for the Health Professions
<www.naahp.org>

Postbaccalaureate Premedical Programs
<www.services.aamc.org/postbac>

Student Doctor Network <www.studentdoctor.net>

Texas Medical and Dental Schools Application Service
<www.utsystem.edu/tmdsas>

Tomorrow's Doctors: AAMC for Students
<www.aamc.org/students>

VirtualEvals <www.virtualevals.org>

Contact Information for Each Medical School

Following is a complete list of contact information for all 130 allopathic medical schools in the United States. It is important to check with each individual medical school to get the most accurate information, as each medical school is different.

Included are the mailing address, phone number, e-mail address, and Web site for each medical school. At the time of publication in July 2009, to the best of our knowledge, all this information was up-to-date and accurate. This information may change over time.

An asterisk * indicates that the school participates with the American Medical College Application Service (AMCAS).

ALABAMA (2)

University of Alabama*
School of Medicine
Medical Student Services
VHP-100, 1530 Third Avenue South
Birmingham, AL 35294-0019
Phone: (205) 934-2330
E-mail: medschool@uab.edu
Web site: medicine.uab.edu/education/prospective

University of South Alabama*
College of Medicine
Office of Admissions
241 CSAB
Mobile, AL 36688-0002
Phone: (251) 460-7176
E-mail: mscott@usouthal.edu
Web site: www.southalabama.edu/com/admissions.shtml

ARIZONA (1)

University of Arizona*
College of Medicine
Admissions Office
P.O. Box 245075
Tucson, AZ 85724-5075
Phone: (520) 626-6214
E-mail: medadmissions@ahsc.arizona.edu
Web site: www.admissions.medicine.arizona.edu

ARKANSAS (1)

University of Arkansas*
College of Medicine
Office of the Dean
4301 West Markham Street, Slot 551
Little Rock, AR 72205-7199
Phone: (501) 686-5354
E-mail: DupuyLinda@uams.edu
Web site: www.uams.edu/com/applicants

CALIFORNIA (8)

Loma Linda University*
School of Medicine
Office of Admissions, 11175 Campus Street, CP A-1108
Loma Linda, CA 92350
Phone: (909) 558-4467
E-mail: admissions.sm@llu.edu
Web site: www.llu.edu/llu/medicine/admissions

Stanford University*
School of Medicine, Office of Admissions
251 Campus Drive, MSOB X3C01
Stanford, CA 94305-5404
Phone: (650) 723-6861
E-mail: mdadmissions@stanford.edu
Web site: med.stanford.edu/admissions

University of California - Davis*
School of Medicine, Office of Admissions and Outreach
4610 X Street, Suite 1202
Sacramento, CA 95817
Phone: (916) 734-4800
E-mail: medadmsinfo@ucdavis.edu
Web site: www.ucdmc.ucdavis.edu/ome/admissions

University of California - Irvine*
School of Medicine, Office of Admissions
Berk Hall, Building 802
Irvine, CA 92697-4089
Phone: (800) 824-5388
E-mail: medadmit@uci.edu
Web site: www.ha.uci.edu/admissions

University of California - Los Angeles*
David Geffen School of Medicine
Office of Admissions, Box 957035
Los Angeles, CA 90095-7035
Phone: (310) 825-6081
E-mail: somadmiss@mednet.ucla.edu
Web site: www.medstudent.ucla.edu/prospective

University of California - San Diego*
School of Medicine, Office of Admissions
Medical Teaching Facility Building, Room 180, Mailcode 0621
9500 Gilman Drive, La Jolla, CA 92093-0621
Phone: (858) 534-3880
E-mail: somadmissions@ucsd.edu
Web site: meded.ucsd.edu/asa/admissions

University of California - San Francisco*
School of Medicine, Office of Admissions
521 Parnassus Avenue, Room, C-200
San Francisco, CA 94143
Phone: (415) 476-4044
E-mail: admissions@medsch.ucsf.edu
Web site: medschool.ucsf.edu/admissions

University of Southern California*
Keck School of Medicine
Office of Admissions
1975 Zonal Avenue, KAM 100-C
Los Angeles, CA 90089-9021
Phone: (323) 442-2552
E-mail: medadmit@usc.edu
Web site: www.usc.edu/schools/medicine/education

COLORADO (1)

University of Colorado Health Sciences Center - Denver*
School of Medicine
Medical School Admissions, Building 500, Room C1009
13001 East 17th Place, Mailstop C297
Aurora, CO 80045
Phone: (303) 724-8025
E-mail: somadmin@ucdenver.edu
Web site: www.uchsc.edu/som/admissions

CONNECTICUT (2)

University of Connecticut*
School of Medicine
Student Services Admissions Center
263 Farmington Avenue, Room AG-062
Farmington, CT 06030-3906
Phone: (860) 679-4713
E-mail: Sanford@nso1.uchc.edu
Web site: medicine.uchc.edu/prospective

Yale University*
School of Medicine, Office of Admissions
Edward S. Harkness Hall
367 Cedar Street
New Haven, CT 06510
Phone: (203) 785-2696
E-mail: medical.admissions@yale.edu
Web site: medicine.yale.edu/admissions

DISTRICT of COLUMBIA (3)

The George Washington University*
School of Medicine and Health Sciences
Office of Medical School Admissions, 2300 I Street, NW
Walter G. Ross Hall, Room 716, Washington, DC 20037
Phone: (202) 994-3506
E-mail: medadmit@gwu.edu
Web site: www.gwumc.edu/edu/admis

Georgetown University*
School of Medicine, Office of Admissions
Box 571421, Washington, DC 20057-1421
Phone: (202) 687-1154
E-mail: medicaladmissions@georgetown.edu
Web site: som.georgetown.edu/prospectivestudents

Howard University*
College of Medicine, Office of Admissions
520 W Street, NW, Washington, DC 20059
Phone: (202) 806-6270
E-mail: hucmadmissions@howard.edu
Web site: medicine.howard.edu/students

FLORIDA (6)

Florida International University*
College of Medicine, 11200 Southwest 8th Street
HLS2-660W2, Miami, FL 33199
Phone: (305) 348-0644
E-mail: med.admissions@fiu.edu
Web site: medicine.fiu.edu

Florida State University*
College of Medicine, Admissions Office
1115 West Call Street, Tallahassee, FL 32306-4300
Phone: (850) 644-7904
E-mail: medadmissions@med.fsu.edu
Web site: www.med.fsu.edu/admission

University of Central Florida*
College of Medicine, P.O. Box 160116
Orlando, FL 32816-0116
Phone: (407) 823-1841
E-mail: mdadmissions@mail.ucf.edu
Web site: www.med.ucf.edu

University of Florida*
College of Medicine, Office of Admissions
Health Science Center, P.O. Box 100216
Gainesville, FL 32610-0216
Phone: (352) 392-4569
E-mail: med-admissions@ufl.edu
Web site: www.med.ufl.edu/oea/admiss

University of Miami*
Leonard M. Miller School of Medicine, Office of Admissions
P.O. Box 016159, Miami, FL 33101
Phone: (305) 243-3234
E-mail: med.admissions@miami.edu
Web site: www6.miami.edu/medical-admissions

University of South Florida*
College of Medicine, Office of Admissions / MDC-3
12901 Bruce B. Downs Boulevard, Tampa, FL 33612-4799
Phone: (813) 974-2229
E-mail: md-admissions@lyris.health.usf.edu
Web site: health.usf.edu/medicine/home.html

GEORGIA (4)

Emory University*
School of Medicine, Office of Admissions
Woodruff Health Science Center Administration Building
1440 Clifton Road, Suite 115
Atlanta, GA 30322-4510
Phone: (404) 727-5660
E-mail: medadmiss@emory.edu
Web site: www.med.emory.edu/prospectivestudents.cfm

Medical College of Georgia*
School of Medicine, Office of Admissions, AA-2040
1120 15th Street, Augusta, GA 30912-4760
Phone: (706) 721-3186
E-mail: sclmed.stdadmin@mcg.edu
Web site: www.mcg.edu

Mercer University*
School of Medicine, Office of Admissions and Student Affairs
1550 College Street, Macon, GA 31207-0001
Phone: (478) 301-2542
E-mail: admissions@med.mercer.edu
Web site: medicine.mercer.edu/admissions

Morehouse School of Medicine*
Office of Admissions and Student Affairs
720 Westview Drive, S.W., Atlanta, GA 30310-1495
Phone: (404) 752-1650
E-mail: mdadmissions@msm.edu
Web site: www.msm.edu/Admissions.htm

HAWAII (1)

University of Hawaii at Manoa*
John A. Burns School of Medicine
Office of Student Affairs and Admissions
Medical Education Building
651 Ilalo Street, Honolulu, HI 96813-5534
Phone: (808) 692-1000
E-mail: mnishiki@hawaii.edu
Web site: jabsom.hawaii.edu/JABSOM/admissions

ILLINOIS (7)

Rosalind Franklin University of Medicine and Science*
Chicago Medical School, Office of Admissions
3333 Green Bay Road, North Chicago, IL 60064
Phone: (847) 578-3204
E-mail: cms.admissions@rosalindfranklin.edu
Web site: www.rosalindfranklin.edu

Loyola University of Chicago*
Stritch School of Medicine, Admissions Office
Building 120, Room 200, 2160 South First Avenue
Maywood, IL 60153
Phone: (708) 216-3229
E-mail: ssom-admissions@lumc.edu
Web site: www.meddean.luc.edu

Northwestern University*
The Feinberg School of Medicine, Office of Admissions
303 East Chicago Avenue, Morton Building I-606
Chicago, IL 60611-3008
Phone: (312) 503-8206
E-mail: med-admissions@northwestern.edu
Web site: www.feinberg.northwestern.edu/admissions/md

Rush University*
Rush Medical College, Office of Admissions, Suite 524-H
600 South Paulina Street
Chicago, IL 60612-3832
Phone: (312) 942-6913
E-mail: RMC_Admissions@rush.edu
Web site: www.rushu.rush.edu/medcol

Southern Illinois University*
School of Medicine, Office of Student Affairs
P.O. Box 19624
Springfield, IL 62794-9624
Phone: (217) 545-6013
E-mail: admissions@siumed.edu
Web site: www.siumed.edu

University of Chicago*
The Pritzker School of Medicine, Office of Admissions
924 East 57th Street, Suite 104
Chicago, IL 60637-5415
Phone: (773) 702-1939
E-mail: pritzkeradmissions@bsd.uchicago.edu
Web site: pritzker.bsd.uchicago.edu/admissions

University of Illinois*
College of Medicine, Office of Admissions
808 South Wood Street
MC-783, Room 165 CME
Chicago, IL 60612-7302
Phone: (312) 996-5635
E-mail: medadmit@uic.edu
Web site: www.medicine.uic.edu

INDIANA (1)

Indiana University*
School of Medicine, Medical School Admissions Office
1120 South Drive, Fesler Hall 213
Indianapolis, IN 46202-5113
Phone: (317) 274-3772
E-mail: inmedadm@iupui.edu
Web site: www.medicine.iu.edu

IOWA (1)

University of Iowa*
Roy J. and Lucille A. Carver College of Medicine
Admissions, 100 Medicine Administration Building
Iowa City, IA 52242-1101
Phone: (319) 335-8052
E-mail: medical-admissions@uiowa.edu
Web site: www.medicine.uiowa.edu

KANSAS (1)

University of Kansas*
School of Medicine, Office of Admissions
Mail Stop 1049
3901 Rainbow Boulevard
Kansas City, KS 66160
Phone: (913) 588-5245
E-mail: premedinfo@kumc.edu
Web site: www.kumc.edu/som

KENTUCKY (2)

University of Kentucky*
College of Medicine, Office of Admissions
138 Leader Avenue Room 118, Lexington, KY 40506-9983
Phone: (859) 323-6161
E-mail: kymedap@uky.edu
Web site: www.mc.uky.edu/medicine

University of Louisville*
School of Medicine, Office of Admissions
Abell Administration Center, 323 East Chestnut Street
Louisville, KY 40292
Phone: (502) 852-5193
E-mail: medadm@louisville.edu
Web site: www.louisville.edu/medschool

LOUISIANA (3)

Louisiana State University - New Orleans*
School of Medicine at New Orleans, Student Admissions
1901 Perdido Street, Box P3-4, New Orleans, LA 70112-1393
Phone: (504) 568-6262
E-mail: ms-admissions@lsuhsc.edu
Web site: www.medschool.lsuhsc.edu

Louisiana State University Health Sciences Center - Shreveport*
School of Medicine in Shreveport, Student Admissions
P.O. Box 33932, Shreveport, LA 71130-3932
Phone: (318) 675-5190
E-mail: shvadm@lsuhsc.edu
Web site: www.sh.lsuhsc.edu/medschool

Tulane University*
School of Medicine, Office of Admissions and Student Affairs
1430 Tulane Avenue, SL67, New Orleans, LA 70112-2699
Phone: (504) 988-5462
E-mail: medsch@tulane.edu
Web site: tulane.edu/som/index.cfm

MARYLAND (3)

The Johns Hopkins University*
School of Medicine, Office of Admissions
733 North Broadway, Suite G-49, Baltimore, MD 21205-2196
Phone: (410) 955-3182
E-mail: somadmiss@jhmi.edu
Web site: www.hopkinsmedicine.org/som

Uniformed Services University of the Health Sciences*
F. Edward Hebert School of Medicine, Office of Admissions
Room A-1041, 301 Jones Bridge Road, Bethesda, MD 20814-4799
Phone: (301) 295-3101
E-mail: admissions@usuhs.mil
Web site: www.usuhs.mil/prospectivestudents.html

University of Maryland*
School of Medicine, Health Sciences Facility I
Office of Admissions, 685 West Baltimore Street, Suite 190
Baltimore, MD 21201-1559
Phone: (410) 706-7478
E-mail: admissions@som.umaryland.edu
Web site: www.medschool.umaryland.edu

MASSACHUSETTS (4)

Boston University*
School of Medicine, Office of Admissions, L-124
715 Albany Street, Boston, MA 02118
Phone: (617) 638-4630
E-mail: medadms@bu.edu
Web site: www.bumc.bu.edu/busm

Harvard Medical School*
Office of the Committee on Admissions, 25 Shattuck Street
Boston, MA 02115-6092
Phone: (617) 432-1550
E-mail: admissions_office@hms.harvard.edu
Web site: hms.harvard.edu

Tufts University*
School of Medicine, Office of Admissions
136 Harrison Avenue, Boston, MA 02110
Phone: (617) 636-6571
E-mail: med-admissions@tufts.edu
Web site: www.tufts.edu/med

University of Massachusetts*
School of Medicine, Office of Admissions
55 Lake Avenue North, Room S1-112
Worcester, MA 01655
Phone: (508) 856-2323
E-mail: admissions@umassmed.edu
Web site: www.umassmed.edu/education

MICHIGAN (3)

Michigan State University*
College of Human Medicine, Office of Admissions
A-239 Life Sciences Building
East Lansing, MI 48824-1317
Phone: (517) 353-9620
E-mail: MDadmissions@msu.edu
Web site: humanmedicine.msu.edu

University of Michigan*
Medical School, Office of Admissions
4303 Medical Science Building I
1310 Catherine Road, Ann Arbor, MI 48109-0624
Phone: (734) 764-6317
E-mail: umichmedadmiss@umich.edu
Web site: www.med.umich.edu/medschool

Wayne State University*
School of Medicine, Medical Education Commons, Suite 322
Office of Admissions, 320 East Canfield Street, Detroit, MI 48201
Phone: (313) 577-1466
E-mail: admissions@med.wayne.edu
Web site: www.med.wayne.edu

MINNESOTA (2)

Mayo Medical School*
200 First Street, SW
Rochester, MN 55905
Phone: (507) 284-3671
E-mail: MedSchoolAdmissions@mayo.edu
Web site: www.mayo.edu/mms

University of Minnesota*
Medical School, Office of Admissions
Mayo Mail Code # 293
420 Delaware Street SE
Minneapolis, MN 55455
Phone: (612) 625-7977
E-mail: meded@umn.edu
Web site: www.med.umn.edu

MISSISSIPPI (1)

The University of Mississippi Medical Center*
School of Medicine
Office of Admissions
2500 North State Street
Jackson, MS 39216-4505
Phone: (601) 984-5010
E-mail: AdmitMD@som.umsmed.edu
Web site: som.umc.edu

MISSOURI (4)

Saint Louis University*
School of Medicine
Office of Admissions
1402 South Grand Boulevard, M226
St. Louis, MO 63104
Phone: (314) 977-9870
E-mail: slumd@slu.edu
Web site: medschool.slu.edu

University of Missouri – Columbia*
School of Medicine
Admissions, Recruitment, and Records Coordinator
Office of Medical Education, MA215 Medical Science Building
One Hospital Drive
Columbia, MO 65212
Phone: (573) 882-9219
E-mail: nolkej@health.missouri.edu
Web site: som.missouri.edu

The UMKC School of Medicine is designed primarily for high
school graduates. Students will earn their baccalaureate and M.D.
degrees concurrently during a six-year program.

University of Missouri - Kansas City (UMKC)
School of Medicine, Council on Selection
2411 Holmes Road
Kansas City, MO 64108-2792
Phone: (816) 235-1870
E-mail: umkcmedweb@umkc.edu
Web site: www.umkc.edu/medicine
      No AMCAS

Washington University in St. Louis*
School of Medicine, Office of Admissions
660 South Euclid Avenue, Campus Box 8107
St. Louis, MO 63110-1093
Phone: (314) 362-6858
E-mail: wumscoa@wustl.edu
Web site: www.medicine.wustl.edu

NEBRASKA (2)

Creighton University*
School of Medicine, Office of Medical Admissions, Criss III
Room 574, 2500 California Plaza, Omaha, NE 68178
Phone: (402) 280-2799
E-mail: medschadm@creighton.edu
Web site: medschool.creighton.edu

University of Nebraska*
College of Medicine, Office of Admissions and Students
986585 Nebraska Medical Center
Omaha, NE 68198-6585
Phone: (402) 559-2259
E-mail: grrogers@unmc.edu
Web site: www.unmc.edu/uncom

NEVADA (1)

University of Nevada*
School of Medicine
Office of Admissions and Student Affairs
Mail Stop 357
Reno, NV 89557-0129
Phone: (775) 784-6063
E-mail: asa@med.unr.edu
Web site: www.unr.edu/med

NEW HAMPSHIRE (1)

Dartmouth Medical School*
Office of Admissions, 3 Rope Ferry Road
Hanover, NH 03755-1404
Phone: (603) 650-1505
E-mail: dms.admissions@dartmouth.edu
Web site: www.dms.dartmouth.edu

NEW JERSEY (2)

University of Medicine and Dentistry of New Jersey – New Jersey
    Medical School*
Office of Admissions
185 South Orange Avenue, Room C-653
P.O. Box 1709
Newark, NJ 07101
Phone: (973) 972-4631
E-mail: njmsadmiss@umdnj.edu
Web site: njms.umdnj.edu

University of Medicine and Dentistry of New Jersey – Robert
    Wood Johnson Medical School*
Office of Admissions, 675 Hoes Lane, Piscataway, NJ 08854-5635
Phone: (732) 235-4576
E-mail: rwjapadm@umdnj.edu
Web site: rwjms.umdnj.edu

NEW MEXICO (1)

University of New Mexico*
School of Medicine, Office of Admissions
Health Sciences Library and Informatics Center, Room 125
MSC09 5085, 1 UNM, Albuquerque, NM 87131-0001
Phone: (505) 272-4766
E-mail: somadmissions@salud.unm.edu
Web site: hsc.unm.edu/som

NEW YORK (12)

Albany Medical College*
Admissions Office, Mail Code 3, 47 New Scotland Avenue
Albany, NY 12208-3479
Phone: (518) 262-5521
E-mail: admissions@mail.amc.edu
Web site: www.amc.edu/Academic/Aboutcollege

Albert Einstein College of Medicine of Yeshiva University*
Office of Admissions, Belfer Building, Room 211
1300 Morris Park Avenue, Bronx, NY 10461
Phone: (718) 430-2106
E-mail: admissions@aecom.yu.edu
Web site: www.aecom.yu.edu

Columbia University*
College of Physicians and Surgeons, Admissions Office
630 West 168th Street, Box 41, Room 1-416
New York, NY 10032
Phone: (212) 305-3595
E-mail: psadmissions@columbia.edu
Web site: cumc.columbia.edu/dept/ps

Weill Cornell Medical College*
Weill Medical College, Office of Admissions
445 East 69th Street, Room 104
New York, NY 10021
Phone: (212) 746-1067
E-mail: wcmc-admissions@med.cornell.edu
Web site: www.med.cornell.edu

Mount Sinai School of Medicine*
School of Medicine, Office of Admissions, Annenberg Building
Room 5-04, One Gustave L. Levy Place, Box 1002
New York, NY 10029-6574
Phone: (212) 241-6696
E-mail: admissions@mssm.edu
Web site: www.mssm.edu

New York Medical College*
Office of Admissions, Administration Building, Room 147
Sunshine Cottage Road
Valhalla, NY 10595
Phone: (914) 594-4507
E-mail: mdadmit@nymc.edu
Web site: www.nymc.edu

New York University*
School of Medicine, Office of Admissions
550 First Avenue, New York, NY 10016
Phone: (212) 263-5290
E-mail: admissions@med.nyu.edu
Web site: www.med.nyu.edu/education

State University of New York University at Buffalo*
School of Medicine and Biomedical Sciences
Office of Medical Admissions
131 Biomedical Education Building
Buffalo, NY 14214-3013
Phone: (716) 829-3466
E-mail: jjrosso@acsu.buffalo.edu
Web site: www.smbs.buffalo.edu

State University of New York Downstate Medical Center*
College of Medicine, Admissions Office, 450 Clarkson Avenue
Box 60, Brooklyn, NY 11203-2098
Phone: (718) 270-2446
E-mail: admissions@downstate.edu
Web site: www.downstate.edu

State University of New York Upstate Medical University*
College of Medicine, Admissions Office, 1215 Weiskotten Hall
766 Irving Avenue, Syracuse, NY 13210
Phone: (315) 464-4570
E-mail: admiss@upstate.edu
Web site: www.upstate.edu/com

State University of New York Stony Brook University Medical
    Center*
School of Medicine, Office of Admissions
Health Sciences Level 4
Stony Brook, NY 11794-8434
Phone: (631) 444-2113
E-mail: somadmissions@stonybrook.edu
Web site: www.hsc.sunysb.edu/som

University of Rochester*
School of Medicine, Office of Admissions
601 Elmwood Avenue, Box 601A
Rochester, NY 14642
Phone: (585) 275-4539
E-mail: mdadmish@urmc.rochester.edu
Web site: www.urmc.rochester.edu/SMD

NORTH CAROLINA (4)

East Carolina University*
Office of Admissions, The Brody School of Medicine
600 Moye Boulevard, Mail Stop 610, Greenville, NC 27834
Phone: (252) 744-2202
E-mail: somadmissions@ecu.edu
Web site: www.ecu.edu/med

Duke University*
School of Medicine
Office of Admissions
Duke University Medical Center, Box 3710
Durham, NC 27710
Phone: (919) 684-2985
E-mail: medadm@mc.duke.edu
Web site: dukemed.duke.edu

University of North Carolina - Chapel Hill*
School of Medicine
Office of Admissions
CB #9500 1001 Bondurant Hall
First Floor
Chapel Hill, NC 27599-9500
Phone: (919) 962-8331
E-mail: randee_alston@med.unc.edu or
    Admis_UNC_SOM@listserv.med.unc.edu
Web site: www.med.unc.edu/admit

Wake Forest University*
School of Medicine
Office of Medical School Admissions
Medical Center Boulevard
Winston-Salem, NC 27157-1090
Phone: (336) 716-4264
E-mail: medadmit@wfubmc.edu
Web site: www.wfubmc.edu/school

NORTH DAKOTA (1)

University of North Dakota
School of Medicine and Health Sciences
Committee on Admissions
501 North Columbia Road, STOP 9037
Grand Forks, ND 58202-9037
Phone: (701) 777-4221
E-mail: jdheit@medicine.nodak.edu
Web site: www.med.und.nodak.edu

OHIO (6)

Case Western Reserve University*
School of Medicine, Office of Admissions, T308
2109 Adelbert Road, Cleveland, OH 44106-4920
Phone: (216) 368-3450
E-mail: casemed-admissions@case.edu
Web site: casemed.case.edu

Medical University of Ohio - Toledo*
College of Medicine, Admissions Office
3045 Arlington Avenue, Toledo, OH 43614
Phone: (419) 383-4229
E-mail: admissions@meduohio.edu
Web site: www.meduohio.edu

Northeastern Ohio Universities*
College of Medicine, Office of Admissions
4209 State Route 44, P.O. Box 95
Rootstown, OH 44272-0095
Phone: (330) 325-6270
E-mail: admission@neoucom.edu
Web site: www.neoucom.edu

The Ohio State University*
College of Medicine, Admissions Committee
155D Meiling Hall, 370 West 9th Avenue
Columbus, OH 43210-1238
Phone: (614) 292-7137
E-mail: medicine@osu.edu
Web site: medicine.osu.edu

University of Cincinnati*
College of Medicine, Office of Admissions
231 Albert Sabin Way, Room E251, MSB
Cincinnati, OH 45267-0552
Phone: (513) 558-7314
E-mail: comadmis@ucmail.uc.edu
Web site: www.med.uc.edu

Wright State University*
Boonshoft School of Medicine
Office of Student Affairs and Admissions
P.O. Box 1751, Dayton, OH 45401-1751
Phone: (937) 775-2936
E-mail: som_saa@wright.edu
Web site: www.med.wright.edu

OKLAHOMA (1)

University of Oklahoma*
College of Medicine, Office of Admissions, P.O. Box 26901
BMSB 357, Oklahoma City, OK 73126-0901
Phone: (405) 271-2331
E-mail: adminmed@ouhsc.edu
Web site: www.medicine.ouhsc.edu

OREGON (1)

Oregon Health and Science University*
School of Medicine, Office of Admissions, Mail Code L102
3181 SW Sam Jackson Park Road, Portland, OR 97239
Phone: (503) 494-2998
E-mail: proginfo@ohsu.edu
Web site: www.ohsu.edu/som

PENNSYLVANIA (7)

The Commonwealth Medical College*
Office of Student Affairs, P.O. Box 766, Scranton, PA 18501
Phone: (570) 504-7000
E-mail: admissions@tcmedc.org
Web site: www.thecommonwealthmedical.com

Drexel University*
College of Medicine, Office of Admissions
2900 Queen Lane, Philadelphia, PA 19129
Phone: (215) 991-8202
E-mail: medadmis@drexel.edu
Web site: www.drexelmed.edu

Thomas Jefferson University*
Jefferson Medical College, Admissions Office
1015 Walnut Street, Suite 110
Philadelphia, PA 19107-5099
Phone: (215) 955-6983
E-mail: jmc.admissions@jefferson.edu
Web site: www.jefferson.edu/jmc

The Pennsylvania State University*
College of Medicine, Office of Medical Student Affairs, H060
500 University Drive, P.O. Box 850
Hershey, PA 17033
Phone: (717) 531-8755
E-mail: studentadmissions@hmc.psu.edu
Web site: www.hmc.psu.edu/md

Temple University*
School of Medicine, Office of Admissions
3500 North Broad Street, SFC, Suite 124
Philadelphia, PA 19140
Phone: (215) 707-3656
E-mail: medadmissions@temple.edu
Web site: www.temple.edu/medicine

University of Pennsylvania*
School of Medicine, Office of Admissions, Suite 100
Edward J. Stemmler Hall, 3450 Hamilton Walk
Philadelphia, PA 19104-6056
Phone: (215) 898-8001
E-mail: admiss@mail.med.upenn.edu
Web site: www.med.upenn.edu

University of Pittsburgh*
School of Medicine, Office of Admissions and Financial Aid
518 Scaife Hall, 3550 Terrace Street
Pittsburgh, PA 15261
Phone: (412) 648-9891
E-mail: admissions@medschool.pitt.edu
Web site: www.medschool.pitt.edu

PUERTO RICO (4)

Ponce School of Medicine*
Admissions Office, P.O. Box 7004, Ponce, PR 00732
Phone: (787) 840-2575
E-mail: admissions@psm.edu
Web site: www.psm.edu

Universidad Central del Caribe*
School of Medicine, Office of Admissions
P.O. Box 60-327, Bayamon, PR 00960-6032
Phone: (787) 798-3001
E-mail: icordero@uccaribe.edu
Web site: www.uccaribe.edu

University of Puerto Rico*
School of Medicine, Central Admissions Office
Medical Sciences Campus, P.O. Box 365067
San Juan, PR 00936-5067
Phone: (787) 758-2525
E-mail: margarita.rivera@upr.edu
Web site: www.md.rcm.upr.edu

San Juan Bautista School of Medicine*
Deanship of Student Affairs, P.O. Box 4968
Caguas, PR 00726-4968
Phone: (787) 743-3038, ext. 236
E-mail: jsanchez@sanjuanbautista.edu
Web site: www.sanjuanbautista.edu/Admissions

RHODE ISLAND (1)

Brown University*
The Warren Alpert Medical School
Office of Admissions and Financial Aid, 97 Waterman Street
Box G-A213, Providence, RI 02912-9706
Phone: (401) 863-2149
E-mail: MedSchool_Admissions@brown.edu
Web site: bms.brown.edu

SOUTH CAROLINA (2)

Medical University of South Carolina*
College of Medicine, Dean's Office, 96 Jonathan Lucas Street
Suite 601, P.O. Box 250617, Charleston, SC 29425
Phone: (843) 792-2055
E-mail: taylorwl@musc.edu
Web site: www.musc.edu

University of South Carolina*
School of Medicine, Office of Admissions
6311 Garners Ferry Road, Columbia, SC 29208
Phone: (803) 733-3325
E-mail: jeanette@gw.med.sc.edu
Web site: www.med.sc.edu

SOUTH DAKOTA (1)

University of South Dakota*
Sanford School of Medicine, Medical School Admissions
414 East Clark Street, Vermillion, SD 57069-2390
Phone: (605) 677-5233
E-mail: usdsmsa@usd.edu
Web site: www.usd.edu/med/md

TENNESSEE (4)

East Tennessee State University*
James H. Quillen College of Medicine, Office of Admissions
P.O. Box 70580, Johnson City, TN 37614-1708
Phone: (423) 439-2033
E-mail: sacom@etsu.edu
Web site: www.etsu.edu/com

Meharry Medical College*
Office of Admissions, 1005 Dr. D.B. Todd, Jr. Boulevard
Nashville, TN 37208-3599
Phone: (615) 327-6223
E-mail: admissions@mmc.edu
Web site: www.mmc.edu

University of Tennessee Health Science Center*
College of Medicine, Admissions Office, Medical Center Plaza
910 Madison Avenue, Suite 500, Memphis, TN 38163
Phone: (901) 448-5559
E-mail: nstrother@utmem.edu
Web site: www.utmem.edu/Medicine

Vanderbilt University*
School of Medicine, Office of Admissions
215 Light Hall, Nashville, TN 37232-0685
Phone: (615) 322-2145
E-mail: pat.sagen@vanderbilt.edu
Web site: www.mc.vanderbilt.edu/medschool

TEXAS (8)

Baylor College of Medicine*
Office of Admissions, One Baylor Plaza, Room N104
MS-BCM 110, Houston, TX 77030
Phone: (713) 798-4842
E-mail: admissions@bcm.edu
Web site: www.bcm.edu

Students applying to any of the following seven allopathic
medical schools must apply through TMDSAS
<www.utsystem.edu/tmdsas>.

Texas A&M University System Health Science Center
College of Medicine, Office of Student Affairs and Admissions
159 Reynolds Medical Building, College Station, TX 77843-1114
Phone: (979) 845-7743
E-mail: admissions@medicine.tamhsc.edu
Web site: www.medicine.tamhsc.edu

Texas Tech University Health Sciences Center
School of Medicine, Office of Admissions, Room 2B116
3601 4th Street, Lubbock, TX 79430
Phone: (806) 743-2297
E-mail: somadm@ttuhsc.edu
Web site: www.ttuhsc.edu

Texas Tech University Health Sciences Center
Paul L. Foster School of Medicine at El Paso
Office of Admissions
5100 El Paso Drive
El Paso, TX 79905
Phone: (915) 783-1250
E-mail: fostersom.admissions@ttuhsc.edu
Web site: www.ttuhsc.edu/fostersom

University of Texas Medical Branch at Galveston
Office of Admissions, 301 University Boulevard
Galveston, TX 77555
Phone: (409) 772-6958
E-mail: tsilva@utmb.edu
Web site: www.som.utmb.edu

University of Texas at Houston
Medical School, Office of Admissions, Room G.420
6431 Fannin Street, MSB G.420
Houston, TX 77030
Phone: (713) 500-5116
E-mail: msadmissions@uth.tmc.edu
Web site: www.med.uth.tmc.edu

University of Texas Health Science Center at San Antonio
School of Medicine
Office of Admissions
7703 Floyd Curl Drive
San Antonio, TX 78229-3900
Phone: (210) 567-6080
E-mail: MedAdmissions@uthscsa.edu
Web site: som.uthscsa.edu

University of Texas Southwestern Medical Center at Dallas
Admissions Office, 5323 Harry Hines Boulevard
Dallas, TX 75390-9162
Phone: (214) 648-5617
E-mail: admissions@utsouthwestern.edu
Web site: www.utsouthwestern.edu

UTAH (1)

University of Utah*
School of Medicine, Office of Admissions
30 North 1900 East, Room 1C029
Salt Lake City, UT 84132-2101
Phone: (801) 581-7498
E-mail: deans.admissions@hsc.utah.edu
Web site: medicine.utah.edu

VERMONT (1)

University of Vermont*
College of Medicine
Office of Admissions
E-215 Given Building
89 Beaumont Avenue
Burlington, VT 05405
Phone: (802) 656-2154
E-mail: MedAdmissions@uvm.edu
Web site: www.med.uvm.edu

VIRGINIA (3)

Eastern Virginia Medical School*
Office of Admissions
700 West Olney Road
Norfolk, VA 23507-1607
Phone: (757) 446-5812
E-mail: nanezkf@evms.edu
Web site: www.evms.edu

University of Virginia Health System*
School of Medicine, Admissions Office
P.O. Box 800725
Charlottesville, VA 22908
Phone: (434) 924-5571
E-mail: medsch-adm@virginia.edu
Web site: www.hsc.virginia.edu

Virginia Commonwealth University*
School of Medicine, Office of Admissions
1101 East Marshall Street
P.O. Box 980565
Richmond, VA 23298-0565
Phone: (804) 828-9629
E-mail: somume@vcu.edu
Web site: www.medschool.vcu.edu

WASHINGTON (1)

University of Washington*
School of Medicine, Office of Admissions
A-300 Health Sciences Building
Box 356340
Seattle, WA 98195-6340
Phone: (206) 543-7212
E-mail: askuwsom@u.washington.edu
Web site: www.uwmedicine.org

WEST VIRGINIA (2)

Marshall University*
Joan C. Edwards School of Medicine
Admissions Office
1600 Medical Center Drive
Huntington, WV 25701-3655
Phone: (800) 544-8514
E-mail: warren@marshall.edu
Web site: musom.marshall.edu

West Virginia University*
School of Medicine, Office of Student Services
Byrd Health Sciences Center
P.O. Box 9111
Morgantown, WV 26506
Phone: (304) 293-1439
E-mail: medadmissions@hsc.wvu.edu
Web site: www.hsc.wvu.edu/som

<u>WISCONSIN</u> (2)

Medical College of Wisconsin*
Office of Admissions, 8701 Watertown Plank Road
Milwaukee, WI 53226
Phone: (414) 456-8246
E-mail: medschool@mcw.edu
Web site: www.mcw.edu

University of Wisconsin*
School of Medicine, Admissions Committee
2130 Health Sciences Learning Center
750 Highland Avenue, Madison, WI 53705-2221
Phone: (608) 265-6344
E-mail: medadmissions@wisc.edu
Web site: www.med.wisc.edu

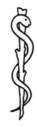